T0369362

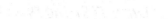

"Career transitions of any kind can be difficult, but when the care of others is included, the value of mentorship increases. With that in mind, Dr. Connie Vance extracts wisdom and knowledge, diamonds and gold, from deep inside the 'mentoring mine.' She clears the pathway for the mentor, as well as the protégé, to understand and participate in this essential relationship. This is a must read no matter where you are in your nursing journey, and especially for nursing students and new graduates."

Carylin M. Holsey, 2010–11 President
National Student Nurses' Association

"Dr. Vance, a leader in the field of mentorship, shares precious gems in her book...with many insights expressed with logic and reason throughout. She guides you through a process of self-discovery as you craft your unique path to the mentors with whom you want to engage and build relationships.... The benefits of mentorship are many as you will discover in her book.... This book will grow with you for years to come."

Barbara Glickstein, RN, MPH, MS
Co-Director, Center for Health, Media and Policy
Hunter College
City University of NY

"This is an empowering and motivating piece. From the perspective of a student nurse, this book will be a guide for students, as well as new nurses, to embrace mentorship and all it has to offer."

Ugo Ogbuagu, RN, BSN (novice nurse)

"Dr. Vance is the guru of mentoring.... She has contributed greatly to nursing by advancing the concept of mentoring relationships to a profession that sometimes has been known to 'eat its young.'...Dr. Vance has provided an excellent resource to nurses as they progress through the various stages of their nursing career. [This book] supports the novice to expert journey and will ensure keeping the best and the brightest in the profession."

Mary Ann Radioli, RN, MA
Director of Nurse Recruitment and Retention
Maimonides Medical Center, Brooklyn, NY

"This is a wonderful book, brilliant and personal, rich in wisdom, filled with emotional insight from shared experiences of nurse colleagues. Connie Vance gives you everything you need to know about mentorship and more."

Donna M. Nickitas, PhD, RN, CEA-BC
Professor, Hunter College
City University of NY
Editor, *Nursing Economics*

"This book demonstrates how valuable it is to seek early and continuous guidance through mentoring as a nurse tries to balance both professional development and skill acquisition in their career.... I think this book should be required reading in Nursing Curriculums."

Athena Palearas, MS, RN, CNN, LNC
Vice President of Education
Fresenius Corporation
Medical Care North America
Waltham, MA

FAST FACTS FOR CAREER SUCCESS IN NURSING

Making the Most of Mentoring in a Nutshell

Connie Vance, EdD, RN, FAAN, is professor of nursing and former dean of nursing at The College of New Rochelle, New York. She has served as a faculty member at New York University, Borough of Manhattan Community College, City University of New York, and Barnes-Jewish Hospital School of Nursing, St. Louis. Dr. Vance holds a doctorate in education from Columbia University, Teachers College, New York; BSN and MSN degrees from Washington University, St. Louis; and a diploma in nursing from Washington Hospital Center, Washington DC. She is a Fellow of the American Academy of Nursing; a Fellow of the NY Academy of Medicine; member of the Nursing Hall of Fame at Columbia University; and honorary member of the American Association of Colleges of Nursing and the Russian Association of Educators of Nursing and Pharmaceutical Colleges. Dr. Vance serves on the NY/NJ Regional Advisory Board of *Nursing Spectrum* and on the editorial review boards of several nursing publications.

Dr. Vance's scholarship, teaching, and writing over four decades have been in the areas of mentorship, leadership development, nursing education and curriculum development, health policy and politics, and global nursing and health. She is a prolific writer, speaker, and consultant to departments of nursing, professional associations, and nursing programs, nationally and internationally, and has received numerous awards for her contributions to nursing education and global nursing. Her publications include *The Mentor Connection in Nursing* (with Dr. Roberta Olson); *The Mentor Connection*; *Mentorship in Nursing Education* (with Dr. Olson); and *Mentorship in Nursing: A Collection of Research Abstracts* (with Dr. Olson).

Dr. Vance is co-founder of the Global Society for Nursing & Health and co-founder of the Nurse Advocacy Forum for Novice Nurses at The College of New Rochelle. She is the recipient of the Nursing Education Award and the Nursing Scholarship and Research Award from Teachers College Nursing Education Alumni Association, Columbia University; and the Humanitarian Award from Hope for a Healthier Humanity.

She continues to be a mentor, teacher, and advocate for nursing students and nurses during her long and distinguished career in nursing and nursing education.

FAST FACTS FOR CAREER SUCCESS IN NURSING

Making the Most of Mentoring in a Nutshell

Connie Vance, EdD, RN, FAAN

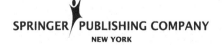
SPRINGER PUBLISHING COMPANY
NEW YORK

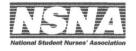

Springer Publishing Company, LLC
11 West 42nd Street
New York, NY 10036
www.springerpub.com

Acquisitions Editor: Margaret Zuccarini
Production Editor: Gayle Lee
Cover Design: Mimi Flow
Composition: Newgen Imaging Systems Ltd.
Project Manager: Ashita Shah

ISBN: 978–0–8261–0689–6
E-book ISBN: 978–0–8261–0690–2

11 12 13 14/ 5 4 3 2 1

The author and the publisher of this work have made every effort to use sources believed to be reliable to provide information that is accurate and compatible with the standards generally accepted at the time of publication. Because medical science is continually advancing, our knowledge base continues to expand. Therefore, as new information becomes available, changes in procedures become necessary. We recommend that the reader always consult current research and specific institutional policies before performing any clinical procedure. The author and publisher shall not be liable for any special, consequential, or exemplary damages resulting, in whole or in part, from the readers' use of, or reliance on, the information contained in this book. The publisher has no responsibility for the persistence or accuracy of URLs for external or third-party Internet Web sites referred to in this publication and does not guarantee that any content on such Web sites is, or will remain, accurate or appropriate.

Library of Congress Cataloging-in-Publication Data

Vance, Connie.
  Fast facts for career success in nursing : makng the most of mentoring in a nutshell / Connie Vance.
    p. ; cm.
  Includes bibliographical references and index.
  ISBN 978–0–8261–0689–6 (alk. paper) — ISBN 978–0–8261–0690–2 (e-ISBN)
  1. Mentoring in nursing. 2. Nursing—Vocational guidance.
  3. Interprofessional relations. I. Title.
  [DNLM: 1. Mentors. 2. Nursing. 3. Interprofessional Relations. WY 18]
  RT86.45.V36   2011
  610.73—dc22   2010026862

Printed in the United States of America by Hamilton Printing Company

Contents

Foreword

In the July 2001 issue of *The American Journal of Nursing*, I wrote an editorial titled "Of Mentorship and Scotch on the Rocks." It was a tribute to the passing of one of my mentors, Anita Golden Pepper, and to her colleague and another mentor of mine, Edna Dell Weinel, both faculty members at the St. Louis University School of Nursing where I received my master's degree in nursing. One of the messages of the editorial was that our most valuable mentors may teach us more about life and living than about our careers. But these mentors also helped me to build a wonderful, productive career by opening doors, providing wise counsel, and raising important questions that they knew I needed to ponder.

I didn't ask them to be my mentors. I think they simply saw that I needed them. Indeed, some of us who have been in this profession for awhile had mentors without knowing that's what they were. I can cite key faculty, clinicians, and colleagues who have helped to shape my career and life without our having a formal mentor–protégé relationship.

In fact, I was privileged to be mentored in political action by the author of this book. I was new to the New York State Nurses for Political Action, an independent political action committee (PAC) for nurses in the state that later became the New York State Nurses Association PAC. Connie Vance and her colleagues at the PAC were smart, savvy nurses who understood the importance of cultivating support relationships with nurses who were new to political work and eager to learn and engage in collective action. Over time we learned from each other, and Dr. Vance referred to these relationships as "peer mentoring" to acknowledge how we can help each other as colleagues to grow and develop.

Another message in my 2001 editorial was that we, as nurses, need to value and embrace mentoring if we're to ensure that we build a new generation of fine nurses who can go beyond what prior generations have accomplished. This book provides students and nurses with a guide to doing so and can be used by protégés and mentors alike. In fact, it could serve as an essential resource for formal mentoring programs that increasingly are becoming a key component of nurse residency programs and nursing education programs.

I might have better used the wise women who were my informal mentors had I known more about mentorship, including how to build a productive mentoring relationship. Dr. Vance's pioneering work on mentorship has provided us with the language, understanding, and strategies for building these essential professional support relationships. This book extends her work in practical and useful ways that will help us build the new generation of excellent clinical experts, advocates, and nurse leaders.

Diana J. Mason, PhD, RN, FAAN
Rudin Professor, Hunter-Bellevue School of Nursing and
Director of the Center for Health, Media, and Policy
Hunter College, City University of New York
Editor-in-Chief Emeritus
The American Journal of Nursing

Preface

Unfortunately, mentoring is still not a common experience for most students and new nurses. They don't know how it works, and how it can benefit them. It is so important to pass the torch to the next generation. There is great longing for mentoring support and belief in us as the future hope of nursing

—A. Hernandez, student nurse

I never had a mentor as a young nurse. At the time, I didn't realize I had been deprived of a special relationship with a mentor, or that I had missed out on something that would have helped me enormously in my career. Upon reflection, it was obvious that I had made costly detours and mistakes, and remembered feelings of self-doubt, confusion, and uncertainty when making critical decisions about my career. I felt sad about missing the chance to share experiences and ideas about my place in professional nursing with a mentor. Much of my career journey was haphazard and serendipitous, and I often lacked essential information and access to networks. I was passionate about nursing and worked hard to be a good nurse, but figuring out things on my own was often difficult and lonely.

Then, in the mid 1970s, when I was examining the concept of leadership in my doctoral studies at Teachers College, Columbia University, my literature search revealed an astonishing fact: that in *every* professional field—*except* nursing—the term "mentorship" was prominent. The word "mentor" was glaringly absent in the language of the nursing profession—it simply was not in nursing's vocabulary. Nurses wrote about preceptors and role modeling, but not mentoring. What did this mean? Did nurses not know about mentoring? Did they not want mentors, or feel they didn't need mentoring? These questions motivated me to include mentoring as a key variable in my investigation of contemporary leaders—the "nurse influentials"—and I made some fascinating discoveries (Vance, 1977). These leaders asserted that they had received substantial mentoring assistance at various points in their careers, and they in turn were mentoring other nurses who were coming behind them. In contrast to the traditional model of having one exclusive senior mentor, the nursing leaders had multiple mentors, who included their peer-colleagues in addition to senior mentors. Indeed, they were quite familiar with mentoring—they had learned, worked, and lived in the presence of strong and abiding mentor connections. The conclusion in my study was that mentors were a vital presence in nursing, particularly among leaders, and that their mentor connections served as an important source of power and influence for them as leaders. My study and subsequent research have demonstrated that mentoring is an *essential* human and professional developmental relationship that empowers and "grows" students, new nurses, and leaders and contributes to their success, satisfaction, and excellence in the profession.

Each and every nurse deserves wise and caring mentors. They deserve to know the presence of the "mentor's spirit—an unseen, affirming influence, and positive energy—a productive, liberating power" (Sinetar, 1998). Nurses give so much to others; they care for people and families in challenging, stressful situations. Nurses are selfless and hard working, and often think they should "go it alone," only reluctantly asking for help. They are also tough and demanding of each other, especially with new and inexperienced nurses. If we would mentor each other more frequently, it would diminish feelings of isolation and uncertainty and create enduring bonds among us for mutual support and encouragement. Nurse mentors can inspire and "champion" other nurses, as well as model and imprint the highest standards of excellence. Mentors empower and affirm us. They can build our self-confidence and bring joy to our work. Through our mentors' presence, our enormous talents and potential can flourish. Nurses have come a long way in understanding and cultivating the mentor concept among their colleagues and students. I believe that "spreading the word" about the necessity of mentor connections will enrich the lives of nurses and students and advance our professional power and influence. When nurses help each other, *everyone* benefits—including our patients.

It is my hope that this practical guide to mentoring—written for undergraduate and graduate students, novice nurses, and the evolving nurse—will contribute to a successful and fulfilling career journey in nursing. I hope that nurses will share the magical gift of mentoring with each other—and that our mentor connections will transform how we learn, teach, work, lead, inspire, and care for each other as we carry out the magnificent, noble work of nursing.

Connie Vance, EdD, RN, FAAN

Acknowledgments

The presence and power of mentoring with my students and colleagues played a central role in the writing of this book. My former and current students and all of the novice nurses entering the profession are my motivation for spreading the Mentor Message. This book is dedicated to them. Their love for nursing and the desire to make a difference in their patients' lives are inspirational. Novice nurses and nursing students need the gift of mentoring that will inform, inspire, guide, motivate, and protect them as they navigate their journey through the amazing world of nursing. It is my hope that the message in this book will nourish them on their journey to professional and personal success and fulfillment.

With deepest appreciation, I acknowledge the generous mentoring of some very special, loving colleagues, friends, and family. Their wise suggestions and guidance during the writing of this book have been enormously valuable. Many of them have been with me from the beginning of my mentoring journey and have been true believers. Others are new friends who appeared in my path on the energy waves of mentoring. I treasure each one of you for your unique contributions: Penny Bamford, Carolyn Castelli, Ethan Ellenberg, Barbara Glickstein, Russell Hullstrung, Deborah Hunt, Auroosa Kazmi, Elaine Larson, Olga Levchenko, Ruth Lubic, Diane Mancino, Diana Mason, Iesha Minors, Donna Nickitas, Ugo Ogbuago, Roberta Olson,

Athena Palearas, Susan Talbott, Russel Taylor, Douglas Vance, Emily Vance, Patrick Vance, Dick Webster, Eileen Williamson, and Launette Woolforde. Also, sincere thanks and appreciation are extended to my editor, Margaret Zuccarini, whom I have dubbed the Mentor Editor for her creativity and cheerleading along the way.

Navigating a Successful Nursing Career

Your Career in Nursing—The Path of the Professional Nurse

Let us each and all, realizing the importance of our influence on others—stand shoulder to shoulder—and not alone, in good cause.

—Florence Nightingale (1881)

INTRODUCTION

You have most likely discovered the unique and rewarding nature of your chosen profession. Nursing provides extraordinary opportunities to make a difference in people's lives. It is most gratifying to be a member of a profession that is held in the highest esteem by the public because of their unfailing trust in us (Gallup Poll, 2009). A career in nursing offers you the profound privilege to serve and care for others. Indeed, your life will be changed and enriched by being a nurse. You will think and act like a nurse through a continually evolving process of education and socialization to the nursing role. Your relationships with others—your family, teachers, mentors,

> colleagues, and patients—will also be a major influence in your development. The partnerships and bonds you establish with mentoring colleagues will help you navigate the path to career success and satisfaction in nursing—to be the best nurse you can possibly be.

In this chapter, you will learn:

1. What it means to be a professional nurse
2. The difference between a career and an occupation
3. The seasons and stages of a nursing career
4. The value of collegiality in a nursing career

BEING A NURSE

Caring for others in health and illness—this will be your life's work as a professional nurse. The work of nursing is exciting, challenging, and always changing. Since the focus of nursing is human beings, every single day in the life of a nurse is special. You will experience the complexity of human beings as you share your patients' most intimate human experiences and make a difference in their lives. You will find the great joy and gratification of serving others in health and illness through the entire continuum of life. Being a nurse calls forth the depths of your humanness and compassion. Inevitably, nursing becomes an integral part of your life and your personal identity.

Professional nurses are expected to expand their knowledge and expertise throughout the different stages of their careers in order to provide safe comprehensive health services to the public in accordance with contemporary best practices. To a large extent, this lifelong learning occurs through collegial relationships with many different people. Mentors are especially significant support people as they can assist you with many essential professional activities as you navigate your career. Mentors guide and advise, inspire and encourage, and open doors to opportunities that will expand your knowledge and expertise. You will be empowered by mentors to become the best nurse you can be—to perform at the very "top of your game."

WHAT IS NURSING?

Nursing is a **profession**, a **discipline**, and a **career**. Various guideposts to nursing knowledge and practice describe the profession, its legal scope, ethical standards, and values. These guideposts are a window into the essence of professional nursing and its societal contract. They remind us that the core focus of nursing is the human being and the human experience of suffering and illness, and wellness and health. As a nurse, you provide care to people through your own humanity in conjunction with professional and ethical standards. Exhibit 1.1 highlights the key elements of professional nursing as described in *Nursing's Social Policy Statement, Code of Ethics for Nurses, Nursing: Scope & Standards of Practice*, and a *State Nurse Practice Act*.

Exhibit 1.1   Guideposts to Professional
Nursing

Definition of Professional Nursing

Nursing's Social Policy Statement (ANA, 2010)
defines nursing as:

> ...protection, promotion, and optimization of
> health and abilities, prevention of illness and
> injury, alleviation of suffering through the diag-
> nosis and treatment of the human response, and
> advocacy in the care of individuals, families,
> communities, and populations.

The International Council of Nursing states
that:

> Nursing encompasses autonomous and collab-
> orative care of individuals of all ages, families,
> groups and communities, sick or well and in
> all settings. Nursing includes the promotion of
> health, prevention of illness and the care of ill,
> disabled and dying people. Advocacy, promo-
> tion of a safe environment, research, partici-
> pating in shaping health policy and in patient
> and healthsystems management, and educa-
> tion are also key nursing roles (http://www.
> icn.org).

Continued

Exhibit 1.1   *Continued*

Legal Scope of Nursing

Each state has a legally authorized Nurse Practice Act that determines the nature and scope of nursing practice within the state. These Practice Acts reflect the obligation of the state, in collaboration with the profession, to protect the health and safety of the public. Every licensed nurse should know the content of the nurse practice act governing legal practice in their state. One state, for example, defines the scope of nursing as:

> diagnosing and treating human responses to actual or potential health problems through such services as case finding, health teaching, health counseling, and provision of care supportive to, or restorative of life and well-being, and executing medical regimens prescribed by a licensed physician, dentist or other licensed health care provider.... (New York State Education Department, 1972).

Standards of Practice and Professional Performance

Nursing: Scope and Standards of Practice (ANA, 2010) guides nurses in the application of their professional skills and responsibilities.

Continued

Exhibit 1.1   *Continued*

The 16 standards comprise:

- **Six standards of practice:** Describe a competent level of nursing care, demonstrated by the critical thinking model, or the nursing process, for professional nurses, advance practice nurses, and nurses in role specialties.
- **Ten standards of professional performance:** Describe a competent level of professional role behavior, related to ethics, quality of practice, education, professional practice evaluation, communication, collaboration, evidence-based practice and research, resource utilization, environmental health, and leadership, including mentoring.

Ethical Guidelines for Nursing

The Code of Ethics for Nurses with Interpretive Statements (ANA, 2001) makes explicit the "primary goals, values, and obligations of the profession" and is a framework for ethical analysis and decision making. "Individuals who become nurses are expected not only to adhere to the ideals and moral norms of the profession but also to embrace them as a part of what it means to be a nurse" (p. 5).

Continued

Exhibit 1.1 *Continued*

The *Code of Ethics for Nurses* serves the following purposes (p. 7):

- It is a succinct statement of the ethical obligations and duties of every individual who enters the nursing profession.
- It is the profession's non-negotiable ethical standard.
- It is an expression of nursing's own understanding of its commitment to society.

WHAT DO YOU DO AS A PROFESSIONAL NURSE?

The nursing profession is complex and holds high expectations for its members to ensure that the highest level of safe, ethical, and quality care is provided to patients and their families. Being an authentic professional nurse requires knowing and being all of these expectations. As a professional nurse you will:

- Possess a specialized body of knowledge
- Provide compassionate patient-centered care
- Uphold nursing's scope and standards of practice
- Employ evidence-based practice in patient care
- Provide safe care within nursing's legal and ethical codes

- Exhibit self-regulation and accountability
- Engage in lifelong study of nursing
- Join professional associations and networks
- Serve as an advocate for patients, colleagues, and yourself

=== *FAST FACTS in a NUTSHELL*

- The focus of nursing is the care of human beings in health, suffering, and illness.
- The nurse's own humanity is central to the nurse–patient relationship.
- Nursing has societal, professional, intellectual, legal, and ethical components.

GET A CAREER: GET A LIFE OF SERVICE

Nurses are privileged to have many opportunities to build exciting careers. Indeed, the nursing profession offers endless possibilities for advancement in specialty practice and leadership roles. Your career success is always just around the corner—if you want it! To "get a career," it is necessary to assess your dreams and goals, examine your dedication and motivation, and commit to active development of your career. To be a professional person is not just having an occupation or holding a job. A career is a lifetime vocation that brings enormous rewards, satisfaction, and self-fulfillment to your life.

A professional career is different from an occupation or a job. A career implies a calling, vocation, or a professional life that provides an essential service to society. A career also offers multiple avenues for personal achievement and advancement. An occupation or a job is daily work or activity that serves as a source of livelihood or income. Whether you view nursing as a profession and career—**or** as an occupation and a job—will determine your personal and professional behaviors and commitment to nursing. Reflect on the profession of nursing and your nursing practice. Some questions to ponder are:

- What does nursing mean to you?
- What are the key values you hold as a nursing student and/or professional nurse?
- What are you most passionate about as a nurse?
- What is your image of the "ideal" nurse that you aspire to be?

Writing down your answers can strengthen your pride in and dedication to your chosen profession. Your reflections can reaffirm your values and ideals in caring for your patients. They can remind you why you became a nurse and the qualities of the nurse you aspire to be.

Table 1.1 illustrates some major viewpoints of nursing as a career in contrast to viewing nursing as an occupation.

TABLE 1.1   Attitudes Toward Nursing as Career Versus Occupation

	Career/Profession	Occupation/Job
Longevity	Lifelong vocation	Temporary; means to an end
Education	University/college	On-the-job and vocational training
Continuing Education	Lifelong and ongoing	Short term; related to job requirements
Commitment	Long term	Varies
Expectation	Extensive professional roles and responsibilities	Reasonable work for reasonable pay responsibilities end with shift

THE CHANGING SEASONS OF A NURSING CAREER

Beginning and advancing your nursing career entails moving through various stages over an extended period of time. This does not happen overnight. The process of professional career socialization is well documented and is similar for every profession. One popular framework, *From Novice to Expert* (Benner, 1984), describes how nurses move through stages of clinical proficiency. The five developmental stages are: **novice**, **advanced beginner**, **competent practitioner**, **proficient practitioner**, and **expert practitioner**.

Successful movement through each stage occurs gradually over time with education, experience, and guidance. Most particularly, active involvement and mentoring by teachers and mentors is a critical element in successfully achieving the tasks of each developmental stage.

Another model of career development highlights the **necessity of support relationships throughout a career,** especially mentoring relationships (Dalton, Thompson, & Price, 1977). This model applies to all professional careers, not just nursing. Table 1.2 illustrates the four successive career stages and the **primary relationships, central activities**, and **major issues** in each stage. You will note that there is a progressive, developmental nature of the activities, tasks, presence of support relationships, and psychological issues in each stage.

The essential value of **relationships** in each stage is emphasized, including the interactions and relationships among mentors and protégés. It is clear that each career stage requires the presence of persons who are committed to being a teacher, mentor, and advocate for you as you move through the developmental steps of growing and learning. These support relationships are particularly important at **transition points**, for example, obtaining your first position after nursing school, getting promoted, deciding on a specialty role, entering graduate study, and changing your workplace setting. At each stage or transition point, you will require different kinds of mentors, depending on your particular goals, needs, and issues. You will need different mentors for different reasons in different seasons of your nursing career to develop your talent for serving others in health and illness.

TABLE 1.2 Four Career Stages

Aspect	Stage I	Stage II	Stage III	Stage IV
Primary relationship	• Apprentice • Novice • Protégé • Learner	• Peer–colleague • Advocate • Mentor	• Mentor	• Sponsor
Central activity/task	• Assisting • Learning • Following directions	• Independent contributor • Specialist • Role model	• Training and teaching • Influencing • Interfacing	• Shaping direction of organization and profession
Major issues	• Dependence • Interdependence	• Independence	• Assuming responsibility for others	• Exercising power and influence

Source: Adapted from Dalton et al. (1977).

════════════════════════════*FAST FACTS in a NUTSHELL*

- The qualities and responsibilities of a professional career are different from having a job or an occupation.
- A nursing career is a life choice and a lifestyle.
- A professional career has distinct developmental and achievement stages.
- Each career stage requires the presence of support people, including mentors.

NURSES NEED EACH OTHER

Nursing is a relationship profession. Nursing cannot be learned or carried out in isolation. Learning about nursing and being a nurse is clearly a "team sport." Enormous interdependence necessarily exists among nurses and nursing students in order to learn and perform the complex responsibilities of nursing. Shared interdependence is central in the relationships among students, teachers, peers, professional colleagues, and leaders. Only nurses can help other nurses learn about nursing. Nurses need other nurses to be important champions and cheerleaders for them as they carry out their challenging work. In order to develop to your fullest potential as a nurse, it is necessary to attract the interest of nursing colleagues and to obtain their mentoring support.

All life and career developmental models acknowledge the central importance of support persons in the life and career journey of every human being. One writer put it this way: "Our survival and development depend on our capacity to recruit the invested attention of others to us" (Kegan, 1982, p. 17). The complexity of a nursing career calls for a substantial support network to ensure your success and satisfaction. It is essential, therefore, that you build relationships with dedicated, caring colleagues who will serve as your mentors and role models. **The bottom line: A successful nursing career requires the support, active involvement, and dedicated investment of other nurses.**

COLLEGIALITY: IT'S A GIVEN

An important aspect of professionalism is called "collegiality." The three "Cs" of collegiality are (1) caring, (2) collaboration, and (3) cooperation. Professional nurses demonstrate collegiality with each other by respecting, mentoring, and advocating for nursing students and nursing colleagues. A high value is placed on collegiality in *Nursing: Scope and Standards of Practice* (ANA, 2004; 2010). Collegial behaviors support the professional development of all nurses as colleagues and include (ANA, 2004):

• Sharing knowledge and skills with peers and colleagues

- Providing peers with feedback about their practice and role performance
- Enhancing professional practice and role performance through interaction with colleagues
- Maintaining compassionate and caring relationships with colleagues
- Establishing supportive teaching–learning work environments
- Modeling expert professional practice
- Mentoring nursing colleagues

The message is clear: if you want to become an excellent nurse with a serious career, be sure to find compassionate and altruistic colleagues. They're worth their weight in gold. When nurses help each other, everyone benefits, including our patients and our profession. If collegiality is absent, and nurses are uncaring and competitive with each other, everyone loses. Nurses are known for their nurturing quality with their patients. This quality must be expanded to include the nurturing of each other as colleagues. Bonding with other colleagues is one of the most important "secrets" in establishing a satisfying professional life. Nurses and students who "live" the standard of collegiality will help create compassionate work environments that are developmental and motivational. Such workplaces will support nurses to become the best they can be through tapping into their talent and potential.

FAST FACTS in a NUTSHELL

- Nursing is a human-focused discipline that requires high-level knowledge, skills, and compassion.
- Nursing is learned and performed in collaboration with others, especially colleagues who serve as mentors, teachers, and role models.
- For career success, build relationships with committed, caring colleagues who will generously mentor you to reach the heights of excellence and satisfaction.

2

What is Mentoring?

I would have become a nurse without my mentor, but never would I have sought the level of professionalism, the degree of compassion, the depth of humor, and the height of empathy that were set as guideposts for me by the conduct of my mentor. The "firsts" of being a nurse are fewer now, but her spirit still prevails.

—Thelma Schorr, RN (1979)

INTRODUCTION

Mentoring is an integral part of life and work. In the nursing profession, it is a collegial partnership that draws nurses and nursing students together as they learn their profession and care for their patients. When nurses champion and cheerlead other nurses— that is mentoring. When nurses open the door of success to other nurses—that is mentoring. Mentoring is a gift of caring and wisdom that nurses give to each other as they navigate the career stages from student to novice to expert. One important outcome of

> *good mentoring is becoming the best nurse you can*
> *be—the blooming of your talent and potential. Every*
> *nurse and nursing student should become acquainted*
> *with mentoring and discover the remarkable ways*
> *that it leads to personal and professional success and*
> *satisfaction.*

In this chapter, you will learn:

1. The historical background of the mentor connection and mentoring relationships in nursing
2. Different types of support relationships and mentors
3. Why and when you need mentors
4. About early career challenges and mentoring

MEET THE MENTOR CONNECTION

Mentoring is an ancient universal reality. It is an integral part of human beings growing up, learning, working, and achieving dreams and goals. Each one of us, whether we realize it or not, has experienced mentoring help from caring people in all the stages of our lives. Mentors are the guides who lead us on our journey. We all need mentors—people who are keenly interested in us and who are willing to guide us in our life and work. For example, families and teachers are important mentors. "Any person lucky enough to have had one great teacher who inspired, advised, critiqued, and had endless faith in her student's ability will tell you what a difference that person has made in her life" (Shenk, 2010, p. 102).

The word **Mentor** was introduced to us thousands of years ago by Homer in the Greek legend, *The Odyssey*. As the story tells it, Prince Telemachus, the son of King Odysseus, was left without the protection and tutelage of his father who was absent from home for 10 years while fighting the Trojan War. Mentor, the trusted friend of the king, was appointed to serve as the prince's guardian, adviser, teacher, advocate, and surrogate parent. In the myth, Athena, the Goddess of Wisdom and Protector of Heroic Men, took it upon herself to assist Mentor, and breathed strength, courage, and wisdom into Telemachus' character. So while the young prince was growing up, destined to become a leader, Mentor-Athena guided, taught, coached, supported, and protected him. This human myth informs us that "Mentor is both male and female, mortal and immortal—an androgynous demi-god, half here, half there. Wisdom personified" (Daloz, 1986, p. 19).

MEET THE MENTOR CONNECTION IN NURSING

> The mentor connection is a developmental, empowering, nurturing relationship extending over time, in which mutual sharing, learning, and growth occur in an atmosphere of respect, collegiality, and affirmation. (Vance & Olson, 1998)

Mentoring has been a "hidden gem" in the nursing profession. Although nurses have mentored each other since the beginning of the profession, including Nightingale's mentoring of several nurses (Lorentzon & Brown, 2003), it is "new" in the sense that the word "mentor" was not widely acknowledged, studied, or implemented in nursing schools, the clinical workplace, and professional nursing associations until the 1980s. Mentoring was notably absent in the nursing literature. This is curious, but understandable, for several reasons. Mentoring was historically a male phenomenon in the older, more established professions. It was not until the late 1970s in American society that women in every field became acquainted with mentoring as they entered male dominant fields in larger numbers. They saw the power of the "old boys network" and male-to-male mentoring relationships. Clearly, mentor connections and networks were integral to the developmental experience of successful career-oriented men. It was even suggested that "everyone who makes it has a mentor" (Collins & Scott, 1978).

Women recognized that without mentor connections they were "out of the loop," as their access to vital information, networks, support, and political know-how was severely limited. Many studies lend credence to the enormous importance of mentors for women's career development and success. More than 400 professional women were surveyed by Collins (1983) who found that although 75% of them had male mentors, they were unsophisticated in seeking mentors, especially other women; and over half of them reported that they "fell into" the relationship and didn't fully comprehend its value.

Historically if women had mentors, they were men. It wasn't until women reached higher positions in the professions, academies, and business that they began to mentor each other.

Since nursing is a female-dominant profession, nurses, along with other professional women, were not historically endowed with experiencing firsthand the career advantages of coaching and moving each other forward through mentor networks. Nurses, particularly as they reached leadership positions, began to realize they were handicapped by the lack of mentors and role models who would coach and guide them in the ways of seeking and sustaining success in their profession. Lacking mentors from the higher ranks of health care, business, and policy arenas, nurses began to mentor each other as colleagues. For example, "The Good Ol' Girls and Collective Mentoring" describes a peer mentoring group that was formed in the late 1970s by several New York nurses to inform and empower nurses for involvement in political action and policy, public speaking, and fund raising (Leavitt & Mason, 1998). One nurse asserts that "Modeling and support by a woman for another woman are important. Male and female experiences differ, and how women do things may be different from men. I think it's important for a woman who has entered a professional field, like nursing, and succeeded, to show other women what it's all about—how to survive and grow in a very paternalistic system."

The reported absence of mentoring in nursing was an enticement to explore this phenomenon. Was mentoring present in any aspect of the profession? Did nurses want and need mentoring? The first formal investigation of mentoring relationships in nursing was conducted by Vance (1977) with a sample of nationally identified nursing leaders, termed the "nurse-influentials." This study, *A Group Profile of Contemporary Influentials in American Nursing*, examined the presence and nature of this collegial relationship among nurses. The major study questions were: Do nurse leaders have mentors? If so, what do mentors contribute to them as individual nurses and to the profession?

The Study Evidence

First, it was found that mentoring relationships were indeed a reality and a significant source of influence and power in the lives of nurse leaders. Eighty-three percent reported having mentors, whereas 93% reported being mentors to many protégés. These leaders were reciprocally receiving and giving mentoring in their various personal and professional relationships, and they attested to the empowerment and self-affirmation they experienced from their mentors. One of these leaders flatly stated that her survival and career advancement were only possible because of her mentors' advocacy and guidance. Her mentors served as role models and a sounding board, gave her courage to take informed risks, and made her feel more confident and secure as she progressed in her work.

Second, these nurse-leaders' mentor relationships were different from classic mentoring relationships. In contrast to the traditional presence of the one all-encompassing, exclusive mentor, the nursing leaders were fortunate to have had several mentors during their career who were nurses as well as other colleagues, administrators, family, and friends. In contrast to most mentors at that time, the nursing leaders' mentors were predominantly female, as would be expected in a highly female-dominant profession. Their mentors included both **expert** colleagues and **peer** colleagues who provided a variety of mentoring assistance to them at pivotal career and decision points. **Different** influences were important at **different** points in their careers.

Third, the nurse-influentials' mentoring relationships contributed to their success as national and international leaders. They, in turn, developed other nurses for leadership roles in the profession. As they had been actively mentored into leadership roles and activities, they mentored the succeeding generation of leaders who subsequently mentored the next generation in a generational legacy. These data demonstrate that (1) those who are mentored become mentors to others; and (2) leaders are "made," not just "born" in an expanding cycle of mentoring networks. The nursing leaders reported that their mentors provided these advantages:

- Served as professional role models for leadership, change, and risk taking
- Were exemplars of excellence in the profession to be imitated
- Provided courage to aspire to "what a true professional nurse should be"

- Instilled self-confidence through belief, trust, and expectation of their success
- Shared the wisdom and power that they had gained from their own mentors

The Study Summary

This study confirmed that mentoring is a vital component of professional nursing and that mentors are essential for nurses' ongoing development and leadership achievement. Further, the profession is elevated as leaders make substantial contributions and changes to nursing and the health care field. It was discovered that not just one mentor, but *multiple* mentors, expert and peer, provided various types of assistance at different points in the leaders' careers. They received mentoring guidance for both professional and personal aspects of their lives and attested to the life-changing role that their mentors played. In turn, they assumed the obligation of mentoring the next generation of nurses and leaders. The mentoring support that the nursing leaders received included:

- Career advice, support, and promotion
- Professional and personal role modeling
- Intellectual stimulation
- Inspiration and idealism
- Teaching, advising, and counseling
- Emotional strength and confidence building

WHAT IS A MENTOR?

Traditionally, the mentor was an older, wiser, more experienced person who guided a younger and/or less-experienced person (the protégé) in a teaching and support relationship during an extended period of time. This is an expert-to-novice model of mentoring. The mentor was usually male and at least 8 to 10 years older than the protégé. In today's world, mentoring is much more diverse—there are no restrictions of gender, age, experience, education, culture, and racial ethnic background. Mentors can be experts and peers, male and female, friends and families. Diversity in mentoring experiences enriches the process. **A mentor is someone who takes a special interest in and actively supports your development. This relationship can develop into an expansive resource of growth, empowerment, and opportunity.**

Real-Life Mentors: A Young Professional Tells Her Story—Auroosa Kazmi, 2010

My mentors have changed my life. They opened doors for me, and encouraged me to imagine a future I could not have seen on my own. I want to be the change for others like my mentors were for me. My boss was my important first mentor. The key was that she cared about me as a person—there was an "emotional connection" on both sides. She saw something in me that at first I didn't see. Her message was, "Go for it! You can be bigger and do more than you realize." Since I deeply respected, admired, and trusted her, her words meant a lot. I began to see that I limited my reach, and she showed me that I could reach higher—that I could be like her, and go where she has gone, and even beyond. My mentor wanted me to achieve and be successful. She had faith and trust in my capabilities, and gave me opportunities to build my skills. This gave me confidence; I was unsure of myself, and she made me feel strong.

My professor is the second important mentor who "discovered" me through classroom work, and suggested that I should study for a master's degree. He asked me some important "life questions": What is meaningful to you as a person? What are you passionate about? What do you want to do in your life? No one had ever asked me such strong questions—they were the "right" questions, and it turned around the direction that I was headed in—to align my decisions with what I really love and want to do in life. My mentor-teacher saw my potential, my capability, and wanted me to take advantage of my potential. His interest and confidence in me reassured me and made me more self-confident.

My third important mentor is a peer and friend. She was going through the same things as me, and urged me to go forward for my master's degree. She said, "Let's do it together." She guided me through the application process and helped me realize that I could do it. Her urging me on and coaching me in specific ways made me believe I could do it and allayed my doubts. I moved ahead with greater assurance. Our sharing has been fun and empowering.

=====*FAST FACTS in a NUTSHELL*

- The mentor connection is a universal human ingredient of growing up, learning, working, reaching for dreams and goals, and realizing potential.
- Mentors are wise guides and champions in your life and work journey who ask you important life questions.
- Mentoring is a developmental, affirming, and empowering relationship that contributes to personal empowerment, achievement, and professional excellence.

MENTORING PARTNERSHIPS IN NURSING

Mentoring has become a popular buzzword in nursing. Information about the mentor concept is being studied and disseminated. Increasingly, nurses like you are experiencing the exciting outcomes of creating new mentoring partnerships with each other. Nurses, acting as both mentors and protégés, are discovering numerous mutual benefits and rewards in these collegial relationships. We know that mentoring enhances safe, high-quality, evidence-based nursing care and strengthens the scientific and research base of nursing. In organizations, mentoring relationships serve as an antidote to disrespectful attitudes and behaviors among nurses and physicians and other health care providers.

Nurses are increasingly mentoring each other in different situations, in many different ways, for various reasons. Both informal mentoring relationships and formal mentor programs are springing up in nursing schools, the clinical workplace, and professional associations. It is important to note that mentoring can occur between novice and expert nurses, between novice and peer nurses, and between expert nurses. For example, a teacher and a student can be fortunate enough to have a relationship in which they **both** teach and learn from each other. Two peer colleagues on a nursing unit, who are **both** novice nurses, can support and guide each other as they learn to become confident and competent nurses. Two nursing leaders can advise and inspire each other, and **both** become more empowered and more accomplished leaders. The current diversity of mentors and protégés provides exciting new opportunities for nurses, as they mutually learn with and empower each other.

Mentoring Partnerships and the National Student Nurses' Association

The National Student Nurses' Association (NSNA) has a long history of promoting mentor relationships among students, faculty, and nursing colleagues, and preventing disruptive behaviors in the workplace. The House of Delegates at the NSNA annual conventions have passed a series of Resolutions indicating their understanding of the power of mentoring support from student to novice nurse (NSNA, *Resolutions*, http://www. nsna.org/Publications/Resolutions.aspx).

Continued

Continued

1996. *In support of the promotion, awareness, and development of mentorship programs.*

2001. *In support of the prevention of workplace violence in health care settings through increased education and awareness.*

2002. *In support of encouraging peer mentorship programs to be incorporated into nursing curricula and/or student nurses associations.*

2006. *In support of increased advocacy for improved preceptor programs to create a robust workforce environment for the nursing profession.*

2006. *In support of professional workplace cultures and decreasing horizontal violence.*

2010. *In support of policy development and increased funding for research on lateral violence in nursing.*

Reciprocal benefits are always present in mentor relationships. Mentoring is not a one-way street. Both mentors and protégés benefit from confidence building, shared connections, ongoing socialization, co-motivation, exploration of new ideas, collaboration in scholarly and research projects, and friendship.

Sharing through mentoring is energizing, fun, and rewarding. It has been suggested that one of the laws of mentoring is the **Law of Fun** (Wickman & Sjodin, 1997). Research has found that when two people are involved in the mentoring process, it becomes an expansive enriching part of their lives. Mentoring adds dimensions of interest and enjoyment. A good mentor relationship is dynamic and creative and gives zest to many aspects of life. Life and mentoring can be fun.

FAST FACTS in a NUTSHELL

- A strong mentor bond develops among altruistic colleagues who generously invest in each other's personal and professional growth.
- Mentoring partnerships can occur between expert and novice nurses, novice and novice nurses, and expert and expert nurses.
- Reciprocal benefits are always present in productive mentor relationships.
- Mentoring, like life, should be pleasurable.

MENTORS PLAY MANY ROLES

The story of Mentor and Athena and their young protégé and the study of the nurse-influentials demonstrate that good mentoring requires a mix of attitudes, knowledge, and skills. Good mentors have the desire, generosity, and experience to invest in the welfare and potential of other people. "...Mentors transcend their own interests, self-promotion and recognition needs, and share their talents with others" (Felton, 1978).

Mentors believe in the dreams of their protégés, hold high expectations for them, and provide opportunities for them to meet those expectations. In another sense, mentors "mold" protégés in their own image as to what they think an excellent nurse should look like. This is **imprinting** the characteristics of what excellence in professional nursing practice should be, and then mentoring for that standard. Mentorship is built on belief, hope, expectation, and unfolding potential as to what things could "look like" and "could be" in the future. **Mentors are "star makers."**

Mentors do many things. Their mentoring activities can be broken down into two categories: (1) career functions and (2) psychosocial functions. Real-life mentors provide all of these in different "doses" at different points in the mentoring relationship. Your mentors can help you with both of these important functions. They overlap and complement each other and will provide you with the full range of mentoring assistance that you need.

Career-focused activities of mentors

- Guide
- Coach
- Network
- Promote
- Open doors
- Teach
- Model
- Protect

Psychosocial-focused activities of mentors

- Affirm
- Inspire
- Cheerlead
- Counsel
- Support
- Advocate
- Empower
- Believe in dreams

═══════════════════════════*FAST FACTS in a NUTSHELL*

- Mentors invest in "futures," "imprint" standards, and "grow their own."
- Mentors believe in and expect great things from their protégés and actively help them reach their potential and achieve excellence.
- Mentors provide a variety of career and personal support activities.

MENTORS, ROLE MODELS, PRECEPTORS, AND COACHES

You will be more confident and better prepared as a nurse when you have strong support relationships with your teachers, peers, and leaders. These relationships contribute important and different forms of guidance, information, and advocacy for you. Developmental relationships can take different forms and differ in their focus and scope. These different roles are described below.

Mentor: A person who provides various aspects of role modeling, precepting, and coaching, but goes above and beyond these. A mentor is like a "professional friend." Mentors invest in both the future development and success of individual nurses, as well as in the evolution of the profession. Mentoring is a freely given gift of interest, time, and involvement.

Role model: Someone who is emulated and imitated as an ideal for superior contributions and achievements. A role model can be admired as your mentor, from afar, and through written work or observed behavior. A historical, influential role model, like Florence Nightingale, is a role model for many nurses around the world.

Preceptor: A specialist or expert who guides the practical training and experience of a student or trainee, usually in the clinical setting. Preceptors are workplace teachers. The preceptor relationship typically occurs during the orientation period and usually does not go beyond the workplace environment in terms of career involvement.

Coach: A trainer or tutor who prepares someone for specific skills or examination. In coaching, the teaching is highly focused and usually occurs between an expert and a novice.

WHY DO I NEED MENTORS?

One novice nurse put it this way: "For me, the essence of my professional being was planted the day I entered nursing school. It was nurtured, nourished, and watered by the wisdom of my mentors. All of the opportunities that came my way through mentoring enabled me to take control of my future and to choose exciting paths in nursing."

A major goal of mentoring is promoting knowledge, skill development, talent, and achievement in a career. It is difficult to hone your talents without the help of others. Mentors find and "polish" the special gifts of their protégés. As human beings, we have evolved to take care of others—we need each other. All of us require the invested involvement of other people to help us develop our talents and to help us be better than we imagined we could. **We need mentors because we can't succeed alone.**

Anecdotal reports and research demonstrate that our professional development and achievement is **easier, faster,** and **more rewarding** when making the journey with mentors. There are many benefits to having the invested support and active advocacy of mentoring colleagues during your career journey. We know that when mentoring is present for nurses, the individual benefits are passed on to the profession and the workplace—to patients, families, and colleagues—and ultimately to the larger society (Exhibit 2.1).

Exhibit 2.1   Benefits of Mentoring

For the individual and the profession:

- Enhanced career success and achievement
- Increased professional and personal satisfaction

Continued

Exhibit 2.1 *Continued*

- Stronger self-confidence and self-esteem
- Preparation for leadership roles and activities
- Talent and leadership development of students and nurses
- Leadership planning and succession
- Empowerment of nurses and the profession
- Sustaining a professional legacy

For the workplace:

- Increased motivation and productivity
- High performance and excellence in practice
- Improved high quality, safe patient care outcomes
- Increased work satisfaction and workplace bonding
- Quality recruitment and high retention rates
- Promotion of a healthy work environment and collegial culture and prevention of disrespectful behaviors that undermine a culture of safety
- Leadership and talent development throughout the workplace
- Cost-saving benefits and outcomes due to above factors

LIVING WITHOUT MENTORS

Is it possible to have a successful nursing career without mentors? Can you develop expertise and find professional fulfillment without mentors? Of course, you can accomplish many things without mentoring assistance. Many people achieve their goals despite the lack of active mentors. Intelligence, ambition, persistence, a good education, and sheer luck are contributors to achievement. Without mentors, however, your career path will be more difficult, uncertain, and lonely. Trying to go it alone entails many mistakes, wrong turns, detours, self-doubt, closed doors, misinformation, and wasted time. Living without mentors is a deprivation of a unique relationship that opens wide the windows of opportunity and the joy of mutual learning and sharing. **The bottom line: Absence of mentors in life and work is a major handicap.**

THE BEST TIME TO HAVE MENTORS

Mentors are a fact of life. They must be present at the beginning of our lives for sheer survival. They then come to us through every stage of our family, personal, and work existence. Mentor relationships begin in our families and have a major impact on gender, role, cultural, and work and career identification and guidance. Throughout childhood and young adulthood, our mentors may include family members, friends, peers, and teachers who are a major influence in school, sports, work, faith communities, and social activities. Then as we move forward in our educational, work, and career endeavors, mentor relationships with our colleagues will provide substantial contributions to our achievement and happiness.

For you, mentors should always be a fact of professional life. Mentors are essential for your full development in every career stage and at professional crossroads and personal transitions. The length of each stage or transition to achieve your goals will depend on your personal qualities, family responsibilities, work setting, education, and life changes. **The bottom line: The best time to have mentors is all the time.**

IN THE BEGINNING—FIND A MENTOR OR TWO OR MORE

During the first few years of your nursing career, it is particularly important to have the guidance and advocacy of involved mentors. The reasons for this are:

- You will be challenged by complex goals and expectations.
- Mentors will help you be more efficient and effective in learning your profession.
- It's more enjoyable (fun) to have people travel with you on your professional journey.

The novice nurse stage starts during the last months of the nursing education program and proceeds through the advanced beginner stage—approximately the first two to three years of your nursing practice. During this time, the new nurse faces specific developmental learning challenges. This is what you will need to accomplish during the beginning years of your career:

- "Learn the ropes" of nursing practice
- Build skills for high-quality, safe performance
- Seek feedback and critique of your performance
- Strengthen your self-confidence and self-esteem
- Move forward with advanced education
- Invest in your nursing career for "staying power"
- Make contributions to your team and nursing unit
- Advance your goals and dreams
- Bond with your colleagues and clinical team members
- Join professional associations for learning, mentoring, and networking
- Become a leader and "make a difference"

In the workplace, in order to provide safe, efficient clinical care as part of a team, the new nurse in the first three years of professional life must learn many things:

- How to **think** like a nurse and **become** a "real" nurse
- Learn from other nurses, doctors, and team members
- Follow the rules of the nursing unit
- Grapple with critical thinking, time management, and delegation
- Provide high-quality evidence-based patient care
- Face ethical dilemmas as an advocate
- Know when and how to ask questions

- Hone verbal and written communication skills
- Practice being a good team player
- Learn the "politics" of the workplace
- Manage conflict and stress
- Care for one's own health and well-being

These are no small feats. Here's where mentors—peer and expert—come in. They can provide important feedback and information, help you see the "big picture," problem-solve with you, and give you valuable survival tips. They are a "sounding board" and will be your advocate, cheerleader, and protector. In other words, mentors are your survival guide and safety net in new and sometimes daunting territory. **Do not travel alone.**

═FAST FACTS in a NUTSHELL

- You need different mentors for different reasons in every season of your nursing career.
- Talent is protected and polished, and leaders are "made" by active mentoring relationships.
- Do not travel your professional journey alone and unprotected. Find caring, competent mentors during your education and throughout your entire professional life.
- When mentoring relationships are present, the empowerment and skill development achieved by the individual nurse will benefit the profession and the workplace—patients, families, and colleagues.

PART

The ABCs of Mentoring

3

Mentoring Begins with "A": Assess Your Mentor Intelligence

It is our belief that through the simple, yet powerful, human phenomenon of mentorship, even one caring, involved, interested person can make a difference in another person's life.

—Vance and Olson (1998)

INTRODUCTION

What you have learned about mentoring can help you develop your motivation and skills in mentor relationships. The first step is examining your career attitudes and goals and exploring how mentors might help you strengthen them. The second step is assessing your readiness and commitment to building relationships with potential mentors. Finding the "mentor match" that works for you and your particular needs is essential. The third step is developing your capacity to enter into mentoring relationships—this is Mentor Intelligence.

In this chapter, you will learn:

1. About the Mentor Readiness Assessment
2. How to determine a good "mentor match"
3. The Mentor Intelligence framework
4. Assessment of your Mentor Intelligence

ARE YOU READY FOR MENTORING?

Only **you** can determine your desire to find mentors. Only **you** can determine whether you are ready to jump into the mentoring pool and swim to success. Finding mentors is not a "given," a matter of "luck," or a gift that falls from heaven. Mentors come into your life **if** and **when** you are ready for them. Mentors will arrive in your professional life **if** you have a commitment and passion for nursing—**if** you have dreams and goals about where you're headed. **Questions to think about: What do I want to be? What do I think I can be? What is important to me?**

It is well known that mentors are attracted to potential protégés because of certain qualities. Curiosity, openness, the desire to learn, enthusiasm, and a strong work ethic are important "attractors." In every field, mentors choose protégés who show promise and potential, share their interests, have career aspirations, work hard, and are motivated to contribute to the profession. Since talent is always a scarce resource, mentors are always on the lookout for it, and go after it. It is not different in the nursing profession. **The bottom** line: **Students and nurses who possess a "career attitude" and positive personal attributes attract the attention of potential mentors. The opposite also holds.**

Becoming aware of how you present yourself to others is important. Whether we like it or not, people notice and make judgments about us, based on the **impressions** we make on them. Therefore, you must honestly assess your attitudes and behaviors to see what they convey. What do you "say" in your attitudes and behaviors? Is your message: "I am a serious professional. I want to learn everything I can about my work, and be the best nurse I can possibly be." Or is your message: "I'm here to do a job. I already know enough about what I'm doing, and I just want to be a good nurse while I'm on duty." These are two very different messages, and the response of colleagues and potential mentors will also be different.

The art of "impression management" is an important key to finding and connecting with people you like and want to be with, including mentors. It is what it sounds like: It is managing the impressions that people have of you (Ensher & Murphy, 2005). Nurses who want to be mentored should take a critical look at the impressions they make on people who could be potential mentors. Reflecting on your "impression management" skills will help you become more self-aware and to honestly assess your behaviors and attitudes and their effect on others. The message of wanting to be the best nurse you can be is a powerful "attractor."

YOUR READINESS FACTOR FOR MENTORING

The first step is to determine if you are **ready** to invest time and energy in a mentor relationship. Remember that first and foremost, mentoring is a personal relationship and requires relationship skills and time. Everything that goes into maintaining good interpersonal relationships also holds for maintaining mentor relationships. Mentoring is a complex relationship involving both personal and professional aspects. Therefore, you have to be ready, prepared, and willing to commit to the relationship and to devote time to it.

The **Mentor Readiness Assessment** (Exhibit 3.1) can increase awareness about yourself and your career. Answering these questions requires careful thought and honest self-reflection. There are no quick and easy answers, and your answers will change as you grow and change. Remember, grappling with self-reflection and self-growth is a lifelong process and should be part of your professional development journey.

Exhibit 3.1   Mentor Readiness Assessment

- Do I want a serious career, or am I satisfied with just holding a job?
- What are my short-term and long-term career goals?
- What is important to me in my profession?

Continued

Exhibit 3.1   *Continued*

- Am I ready to make a serious commitment to career success?
- Am I willing to take the initiative and devote time and energy to advance my career and self-development?
- Am I willing to ask for help, and accept advice and feedback?
- Do I have what it takes to be a leader?
- Am I curious and committed to lifelong learning and development?
- Can I be open and honest with myself and others?
- Do I want mentors? For what reasons?
- Am I willing to invest time and energy in mentor relationships?

Writing your answers to this assessment in a journal is helpful in reflecting on this information and reviewing your attitudes and feelings over time. Journaling provides a great growth opportunity for self-review and examination of developmental changes in your professional attitudes and behaviors. Recording perspectives in a journal can be a springboard for gaining self-knowledge and confidence in nursing practice (Billings & Kowalski, 2006). Discussing your Mentor Readiness Assessment in a class or seminar, and with a friend, colleague, or family member is recommended.

A VISION OF MENTORS—WHAT ARE YOU LOOKING FOR?

If you decide that mentors are for you, it is a good idea to create a snapshot of what your "ideal" mentor would look like. Some useful questions to guide you are: What specific talents and interests do I want to develop? What do I want to achieve through a mentoring relationship? What qualities of a mentor are a "fit" with my personality and my needs and goals? What kinds of help will I need?

Since it takes two people—the mentor and the protégé—to create a mentoring relationship, each relationship will be unique and different, depending on the personal qualities of the two people. At the very least, there must be **mutual respect**, **trust**, and **interest** in each other for the formation of a successful "mentor match." **Faith** and **belief** in each other fuel the relationship. **Similar values and goals** as well as **shared interests** are also "attractors." Some mentor relationships have a sort of chemical attraction, and there is an emotional investment in each other.

A snapshot of your "ideal" mentor will look different than anyone else's because of your unique personality and goals. Research, however, has shown that excellent mentors possess some basic traits that promote successful mentoring outcomes. These qualities reflect the art of mentoring and will be present in the excellent mentor. Six of these traits are: (Johnson & Ridley, 2004)

Traits of Excellent Mentors

Generosity of spirit—Unselfish, not self-centered, or a "queen bee"

Self-confident—Knows, respects, and likes self; is not threatened by other people's achievements

Competent—Has an area of expertise that is recognized; is knowledgeable and productive

Open to mutuality—Is willing to share ideas and information and engage in give-and-take

Trustworthy—Has high integrity, honesty, keeps promises, and maintains confidentiality

Empathic—Possesses emotional intelligence and high-level interpersonal, communication, and listening skills

Jot down in your journal or notebook what your "ideal" mentor looks like and the qualities that would appeal to you as a protégé. This list will help you focus your search for the "right" mentoring partners.

FAST FACTS in a NUTSHELL

- Your readiness factor for mentoring is a major determinant to jumping into the mentor pool.
- Attracting mentors who are willing to invest in your personal and professional growth depends on your personal qualities and the "impression messages" you send.
- Find the right "mentor match" with persons who have qualities that are a good "match" with your unique personal and career goals and needs.

MENTOR INTELLIGENCE

Several forms of intelligence make up your potential for achievement and success. Your cognitive intelligence (IQ) and emotional intelligence (Goleman, 1995) are vital ingredients in your toolkit for success. Current research and thinking posit that IQ—intellectual "horsepower"—is a threshold competence to enter a professional field, but does not necessarily make one a star. Emotional intelligence, on the other hand, is necessary to go beyond the beginning threshold and reach the potential of one's talents. This type of intelligence is the driver for superior performance and the emergence of exceptional leadership.

The Power of Mentor Intelligence

I suggest a third type of intelligence—**mentor intelligence**—that can provide a huge advantage for advancing personal and professional achievement. **Mentor intelligence is the capacity for entering into mentoring relationships.** It is the ability to give and receive mentoring that can enhance the development of your personal talents and untapped potential. This capacity to enter into mentoring relationships applies to both being a mentor and a protégé.

Mentor intelligence has three characteristics or competencies:

- **Mentoring mentality.** Knowing the theory and process of mentoring. Acquiring knowledge about mentoring through study, self-reflection, and experience.

- **Mentoring lens.** Viewing students, colleagues, and yourself as deserving of the multiple benefits of mentoring. Having "intentionality" to give and receive mentoring in different relationships.
- **Mentoring momentum.** Possessing personal qualities that enable you to create and sustain mentor relationships. "Living" mentoring as an attitude and lifestyle in both mentor and protégé roles.

Assess your mentor intelligence by completing the **Mentor Intelligence Checklist** (Exhibit 3.2). Review your mentoring activities in light of the three aspects of mentor intelligence. **The bottom line: Your mentor intelligence "score" is a snapshot of the presence, quantity, and quality of your mentor connections.**

Exhibit 3.2   Mentor Intelligence Checklist

Presence of mentors: yes ___ no ___
Presence of protégés: yes ___ no ___
Number of mentors: ___
Number of protégés: ___
Quality of mentoring activity (describe your mentor relationships):
Longevity: _____
_____

Continued

Exhibit 3.2 *Continued*

Frequency of interactions: _____

_____

Honesty and openness: _____

_____

Goals and activities: _____

_____

Shared projects: _____

_____

Other key aspects: _____

_____

Your mentoring mentality: (describe) _____

_____

Your mentoring lens: (describe) _____

_____

Your mentoring momentum: (describe) _____

_____

Mentor intelligence can make significant contributions to empowerment and leadership in the nursing profession, in addition to the individual benefits that you and other nurses will find. Mentor intelligence can:

• Develop the knowledge, skills, and talents of each student and each nurse

- Promote a "culture of collegiality" throughout the profession
- Create humanistic nursing educational environments that support the developmental path of students and nurses
- Cultivate compassionate, respectful clinical work environments that nurture and polish the gifts of every person who works in them
- Contribute to provision of safe, high quality, and humane nursing care to patients and families
- Expand the leadership talent pool in the nursing profession and the health care system

FAST FACTS in a NUTSHELL

- Mentor intelligence consists of three competencies: mentoring mentality, mentoring lens, and mentoring momentum.
- Every student and every nurse should develop mentor intelligence for talent development and career achievement.
- The outcomes of mentor intelligence benefit the individual (you), your patients and their families, the nursing profession, and the workplace.

4

The "B" of Mentoring: *Build* Your Mentor Connections

I have a mental picture of my mentor opening a door for me. At times it felt as if she had to push me through the door, but eventually, I journeyed to a different place, and I will never be the same again. My mentor treated me as if I had potential and as an equal. She challenged me and led me through the first door of success, and that was all I needed. Ever since then, I have known my direction in life and have followed it, despite obstacles.

—Melissa Charlie (1998)

INTRODUCTION

If you want to navigate your professional journey accompanied by mentors, you need to have a destination (goals) and a roadmap (a plan). Goals and a plan will guide your search for good travel partners. Sometimes, serendipity and chance produce mentors. A potential mentor may appear along the way due to unforeseen circumstances and opportunities. At the same time, having a plan in mind solidifies your intent

> *to build mentor bonds and provides ideas about getting from "here to there." Finding and selecting a variety of mentors will be an important part of your action plan.*

In this chapter, you will learn:

1. How to create a Personal Mentor Action Plan
2. Types of mentors and where to find them
3. Selection process of the mentor and the protégé
4. How to inventory individuals and groups as potential mentors

GETTING STARTED

Start with the data from your **Mentor Readiness Assessment** (Chapter 3, Exhibit 3.1). If you have decided that you: (1) want to have a serious career in nursing; (2) are ready to look for mentors who will invest in you and your career; and (3) are willing to commit some time and energy to mentor relationships, then you are ready to create an Action Plan for Career Success.

CREATE YOUR PERSONAL MENTOR ACTION PLAN FOR SUCCESS

A plan will provide you with useful guideposts as you begin your mentoring journey. Beginning a working draft of your plan will most likely produce ideas you hadn't thought of before. Planning will also encourage you to take the initiative to build new mentor connections, in addition to the mentors you already have. The elements of this Action Plan are: (1) vision and goals, (2) mentoring strategies, (3) implementation activities, and (4) mentoring outcomes. The **Personal Mentor Action Plan** is in **Appendix A**.

First, begin to fill in this Plan. This will require thinking and working on it over several sessions and, of course, on an ongoing basis. Second, review it and reflect on your answers. Make changes and add new ideas. The next step is to use this Plan as a guide as you move forward in your career. Remember that your professional needs and strategies are always changing as you proceed through various stages and transitions. Reviewing and revising your plan will be necessary as you advance your career and personal life. Some transitions include getting your first position, changing your workplace, going to graduate school, deciding on a specialty area of practice, relocating, being promoted, and having a family. Your plan is a dynamic work-in-progress—like you—that will evolve as you progress in your life and career. A description of the four components of the **Personal Mentor Action Plan** follows:

Professional Vision and Goals: A professional *vision* describes your dreams and ambitions—the big picture of what you want to do and where you want to go in your career. What excites you about nursing? What is important to you as a nurse? What do you want to be? What do you want to contribute to your patients and your profession? Your *goals* are the ways to reach your career vision.

Goals might include deciding on the specialty practice that excites you; preparing for the types of practice roles and work positions that you envision; obtaining advanced education; getting specialty certification; and participating in professional nursing associations.

Mentoring Strategies: These are the "how's" of reaching your goals. Strategies might include identifying ways to locate your "ideal" mentors, listing the names and/or roles of potential mentors, and specifying approaches to choosing and/or being chosen in mentor relationships. You may already have mentors, and you can pinpoint how to nurture these mentor connections.

Implementation Activities: This is jumpstarting your mentoring activities; that is, activating the strategies, with time lines, to reach your vision and goals. These should include both individual and/or collective avenues. Examples are joining a formal mentor program in nursing school or your workplace, contacting a nurse whom you admire and would like to learn from, joining a nursing association, networking at your workplace, and meeting more frequently with your current mentors. Specify a time target for each approach. Which approaches are short term, long term, or a combination of both? Who are specific persons you plan to meet? Who can help you with particular aspects of implementing your strategies?

Mentoring Outcomes: This is reflection and review of what you have achieved and what accomplishments are in progress in relation to the goals, strategies, activities, and time frames that you specified. These mentoring outcomes will reflect the development of your **Mentor Intelligence**. As you cultivate a mentoring mentality, enhance your mentoring lens, and create mentoring momentum, you will be on your way to building mentor connections that will help you become an excellent nurse and achieve your goals. Ongoing review and achievement of specific goals, strategies, and activities will guide the revision of your plan. Revisit this plan at intervals of three to six months.

WHERE ARE ALL THE MENTORS?

As you develop strategies in your mentor action plan, it helps to know where good mentors can be found. In truth, mentors are **everywhere**—in schools, hospitals, professional associations, clubs, community groups, religious centers, and political organizations. Potential mentors can be found at your workplace, conferences, classrooms, clinical units, meetings, and conventions. Wherever like-minded professionals and students meet and mingle with each other, there is a mentor goldmine.

Creating your mentor networks can happen anywhere. Getting "out and about" and being involved in different activities and events is how you **gain access** to potential mentors. You can't just go to your work unit with the same people, day in and day out, and expect to find new and diverse mentors. You have to find ways to move out of your comfort zone to experience new people and new opportunities. Just around the corner may be an excellent mentor or two...but you have to be "out there" to bump into them, and for them to find **you**. You can also find mentors through online social networking platforms.

Access to potential mentors is facilitated through electronic networks. **The bottom line: Develop a detective's eye for finding mentors. Strategize about** *how* **and** *where* **you and your mentors can locate each other.**

════════════════════════*FAST FACTS in a NUTSHELL*

- Creating a Personal Mentor Action Plan is a major step in creating mentor connections.
- Your Personal Action Mentor Plan consists of your professional vision and goals, mentoring strategies, implementation activities, and mentoring outcomes.
- Mentors are everywhere. Be on the lookout for potential mentors by activating your Mentor Intelligence. Also nurture your current mentoring relationships.

"CHOSEN" AND "MATCHED" MENTORS: PUT BOTH TO WORK FOR YOU!

Two main types of mentor relationships will boost your career development: (1) relationships that are "chosen" by the mentor and protégé, and (2) relationships in which mentors and protégés are "matched" or assigned in a formalized program. It's a good idea to have both types of mentors in your repertoire, as each offers different opportunities and benefits. Look for both for a well-rounded mentoring experience.

Mentors and Protégés—By Choice

Mentors and protégés usually choose each other by virtue of having a "natural" affinity for each other for various personal and professional reasons. This type of mentor relationship is fueled by mutual attraction or "chemistry," a reciprocal emotional connection, common interests and goals, mutual admiration and trust, and enjoyment of one another's company. This is a mentoring model in which two persons make a positive impression on each other and commit to share and work together in various ways. As one protégé describes it, "My mentor and I had an emotional connection. She genuinely cared about me as a person and wanted me to be successful, and I deeply admired and trusted her, and wanted to succeed to justify her faith in me. Our relationship has changed over time, but the initial connection is still there. It's life changing and hard to describe."

This traditional mentoring model exists between expert and novice and between peer and peer. It can be short term or long term, depending on the goals, needs, availability, interests, and personal factors of the individuals. This "chosen" relationship is unique and special; it happens between people who "click." And it entails a personal and time commitment to each other.

Mentors and Protégés—By Match

This is a planned organizational model in which mentors and protégés are formally selected, "matched," and assigned to each other in a collective setting, such as a school, hospital, corporation, or professional association. This approach assists people through a formal process to find organizational mentoring partners who may have similar interests and goals in their profession and/or organization. Chemistry and mutual attraction may or may not be present; the "holding glue" is respect for and interest in each other as like-minded professionals. These "matched" mentor connections can involve a formal expert-to-novice relationship, such as in an orientation or mentorship program for novice nurses or newly hired nurses in a nursing department. It can also exist in a formal peer-to-peer relationship, such as in a student-run mentor program in a nursing school. However, the formal "assigned" mentor is more typically a senior, experienced person mentoring a novice, or less-experienced person. "Assigned" mentors are found in on-the-job mentor programs, professional associations, specialty nursing organizations, and community volunteer programs. The time limits of these relationships are spelled out in an informal contract and are usually short term and renewable, if desired. The formal method of matching mentors and protégés is efficient and effective in linking people; however, it has unique challenges of "fit" and personal affinity.

There are numerous examples of formal mentorships in the nursing profession. In the clinical workplace, these mentorships can occur in staff orientation programs; preceptor/mentorship programs for students; nurse residency programs, clinical internships and externships; and clinical specialty programs. In nursing schools, mentor programs may link different levels of students; match alumni with undergraduate or graduate students; and establish mentor matches through student organizations. Currently, professional nursing and student associations are very proactive in offering formal mentor programs that address their members' needs in various ways. These relationships provide numerous developmental, networking, and advocacy benefits to both the individual member and the association. A selection of collective mentoring opportunities is listed in **Appendix B: Resources for Collective Mentoring and Networking.**

WHO CHOOSES WHOM?

Traditionally, mentors chose their protégés. This is the model in which senior, experienced, and established persons choose students, neophytes, or "rising stars" whom they then assist on their career path. This method of choosing a protégé is still considered the "gold standard" of classic traditional mentoring. There are stories in every field about someone being "chosen," taken "under the wings" of a mentor, and the subsequent rising of that chosen protégé to unexpected heights of success. This relationship is often transformative and becomes a major influence in the lives of both mentor and protégé.

> Mentoring strikes a universal chord. If we're lucky, we have met that inspiration that challenged us to be better, or try something new (Dalton, 2010).

Nurse managers, leaders, and teachers are strongly encouraged to identify and "go after" students and nurses with talent, expect them to succeed, set a high standard for their educational and clinical performance, and mentor them for achievement and success. This is a powerful human resource approach that assures a continuous supply of committed and competent nurses and effective leaders in the profession.

On the other hand, students and new professionals are strongly encouraged to "take the initiative," to assess their dreams and goals, and to "go after" and choose people whom they admire and trust, want to emulate, and could help them thrive and excel. Actively seek out mentors. They tend to be busy people, and may simply overlook someone who has talent and potential. Dig for the "gold mine" of great mentors who can help you blossom into a high-performance nurse and leader.

The Voice of a Novice Nurse

My dream was to specialize in migrant nursing, as I came from a family of migrant workers and wanted to improve their health care. At a nursing conference I heard a high-level nurse speak about her research in migrant nursing, and it was thrilling. I really wanted to speak with her, but I felt too shy. I kept her in my mind, but didn't have the courage to reach out to her. However, at another nursing conference, I met a nurse who spoke about mentoring, and I told her about my dream to meet my "role model." She said, "You should really contact her. Migrant nursing is her passion, and she would undoubtedly be happy to talk with a young nurse who wants to follow in her footsteps. She might be just the mentor you're looking for. Go for it." After careful thought for several weeks, I decided to take the leap, and I called her, and she was thrilled to hear from me. I couldn't believe it—here I was, a new nurse talking to an important leader, saying she would help me in any way! She has become my mentor in the specialty I love so much, and has supported and guided me in so many ways. I am so happy that I finally reached out to her. She has been an inspiration and set me on my path to realizing my dream.

Who chooses whom is not as important as **making mentoring happen**. Having a **mentoring mentality** and a **mentoring lens** everywhere you go greatly improves your chances of finding mentors and finding persons whom you can mentor. This is creating your **mentoring momentum**. Remember that there is always someone ahead and behind you in your education, work, and career, so that numerous opportunities exist for mentoring by "choice" and through mentor "matching" programs.

FAST FACTS in a NUTSHELL

- Mentors are found in two ways: by "choice" of the mentor and protégé, and by "match" or assigned mentoring.
- Mentors can choose you, and you can take the initiative to choose your mentors.
- Make mentoring happen by raising your Mentor Intelligence. Develop a mentoring mentality, mentoring lens, and mentoring momentum.

IDENTIFYING YOUR MENTOR POOL

Whether you are "chosen," the "chooser," and/or "matched," it is important to identify the individuals and groups in your current and future networks and to assess how they might assist you with your career goals. The **Inventory of Mentor Networks** (Exhibit 4.1) can help you strategize about strengthening current mentor relationships, as well as developing new contacts. This Inventory provides a map of where you're at and where you plan to go with mentors. Answer the questions in this Inventory. Your answers will add useful information to your **Personal Mentor Action Plan in Appendix A.**

Exhibit 4.1   Inventory of Mentor Networks

1. Name five key **people** in your network of peers, colleagues, mentors, friends, and family.
2. Describe why each **person** is so important to you, using specific adjectives and examples.
3. Who are additional **persons** you would like to include in your network? Why?
4. List the **groups** you belong to (professional, school, work-related, social, community, etc.).
5. Describe what you get from these **groups** (ideas, information, contacts, social life, support, etc.).
6. What additional **groups** would you like to belong to? Why?

Continued

Exhibit 4.1 *Continued*

7. What are your **ambitions and career goals**? Which of these do you want to achieve within the next two years? The next five years?

8. **Who and what could help you** in attaining your goals? (include your personal qualities, peer–colleague network, mentor connections, group networks, friends, family)

9. **How can I help students and my colleagues** build their mentor networks?

FAST FACTS in a NUTSHELL

- Make an inventory of current and potential support persons and groups in your network who could help you attain your career goals.
- Identify how you can help students and colleagues build their mentor networks through your network.
- Remember that mentoring and networking are reciprocal in nature. Be on both the giving and receiving ends.

5

The "C" of Mentoring: *Cultivate* Your Potential and Talent for Success

Human potential remains a mystery. It is often stifled— a great and common tragedy. Our society badly needs organizations and people who will help each other move relentlessly toward realizing their potential.

—M. De Pree (1997)

INTRODUCTION

Success doesn't just happen. Personal qualities, family, environment, preparation, hard work, and serendipity all play a role. But the most important element is YOU. You create your own success—or not. You are in the driver's seat. The winning formula is to invest thought, time, and attention to your nursing career. Think about what you want to do in your career, look for opportunities, and seize them. Having a serious career commitment and a keen desire to learn will attract the attention of others, including mentors, who will guide you along your

> *path. Their advocacy will be a major factor in the unfolding of your potential and talent and your life and professional success.*

In this chapter, you will learn:

1. About success and factors leading to success
2. Cultivating your potential and talent through Mentor Intelligence
3. How to be a "perfect" protégé
4. The difference between mentoring and "tormenting" behaviors
5. About mentoring cultures: "places of realized potential"

YOU + OTHERS = SUCCESS

What is success? "Success" is a complex phenomenon. Everybody has their own idea of what it is and what it means to them. Generally, it is something achieved that is desired or intended. Success can be internal and external. In other words, the meaning of success depends on what the person, the environment, and the culture says it is. What does success mean to you? What does success mean to the people around you—your family, teachers, and peers? What are your dreams of success? What drives you to succeed—to want to work at the "top of your game"?

In the bestseller, *Outliers*, Gladwell (2008) claims that successful people, or "outliers," are markedly different from other people in achievement. He points out that success does not just happen due to individual merit. Outliers do *not* achieve success alone. Successful people are unique products of their history, parentage, opportunity, support, and legacy. Success in one's field requires individual talent, hard work, drive, passion, and other people's belief and assistance. Success, says Gladwell, is "grounded in a web of advantages and inheritances, some deserved, some not, some earned, some just plain lucky." Becoming a successful nurse, athlete, lawyer, musician, chef, or entrepreneur—the success factors are the same: a hodgepodge of individual, collective, and environmental forces.

YOU + OTHERS = SUCCESS IN NURSING

Success in nursing depends on **you** plus **others**—the people you surround yourself with. It is as simple and as complex as that. The "**you factor**" is a mixture of your passions, motivation, and determination to be an excellent nurse, preparation (education and deliberate practice), and seizing opportunities that come your way. In addition to obtaining a solid education, preparation includes the "work hard" factor. Hard work and "deliberate practice" distinguish those who rise to the top of their fields (Coyle, 2009). Successful people simply work much, much harder than everyone else. Gladwell invokes the "10,000-hour rule" as the magic number of greatness. This is the number that researchers have identified as the investment of time one must make in order to achieve high-level expertise. For nurses, who usually work about 2,000 hours a year, this would be the equivalent of at least five years of consistent, focused practice. Practically speaking, becoming an expert nurse, or an expert in any area or any field, requires at least 5 to 10 years of educational preparation, experience, and focused, "deliberate practice." "It seems that the brain takes this long to assimilate all that it needs to know to achieve true mastery," writes neurologist, Levitin (2006).

The "**other factor**" in your success formula includes those individuals in your circle of family, friends, and colleagues who are your "cheerleaders" and "champions"— who believe in you and expect you to succeed, and are willing to promote you and your dreams by providing challenging work and learning opportunities. This is where mentoring enters in as one of the decisive success factors in life and work. No one succeeds alone, and mentors are your "keys" and "door openers" for achieving success. Mentors can field you the tough questions, help you see the big picture, provide learning experiences, and offer important feedback and suggestions.

The **Inventory of Mentor Networks** (Exhibit 4.1) in Chapter 4 provides a framework for you to describe the individuals and groups in your network who are currently helping you as personal and career mentors, as well as individuals and groups who could be significant contributors to your goals in the future. Becoming a successful nurse takes **talent**, **time**, and a **team**! Make sure that mentor connections are a major ingredient in your personal team.

SUCCESS AND TALENT: DISCOVER IT AND DEVELOP IT

Talent is a precious thing. It consists of your unique innate abilities. Your talent is your potential and power—your capacity to learn, perform, and achieve. Recent studies about talent suggest that it is a process, rather than a cut and dried statistical factor in achievement (Shenk, 2010). Factors that unlock talent include perseverance, passion, self-confidence, and discipline. Convincing yourself that your potential and talent are probably greater than you realize is a big step. Novice professionals sometimes don't set their sights high enough and limit their reach. Other people—including mentors and teachers—can often see your capabilities before you see them. Talent doesn't magically emerge—it is often hidden potential, lying in wait to be ignited. Like success, talent develops as a combination of many personal, interpersonal, and external factors.

Do you know what **your** talents are? Do you know what you want to be, and who you think you can be? Take stock. You most likely know what you have a talent and "flair" for doing—what you love and enjoy—those things that you are passionate about and drive you—that others tell you that you shine at. Self-reflection and evolving self-awareness can give you confidence and motivation to pursue your talents. Unleashing potential and talent requires a curious mind and openness to unexplored opportunities and possibilities. This includes active searching for mentors in many different places.

Mentors can provide an important reality check by their belief and faith in you and your potential. They often can see emerging strengths that you cannot see—they can help you see the "big picture." Mentors are a "spark"—they can wake you up to bigger possibilities and bigger dreams. They will ask you the big Life Questions—they will tell you what you **need** to hear, in contrast to what you **want** to hear. Their teaching, guidance, and coaching will help identify and nurture your talents. **The bottom line: Unfolding of potential and talent requires help from caring colleagues, family, and friends, combined with your hard work and determination.**

===*FAST FACTS in a NUTSHELL*

- Success comes from a mixture of "you" and "other" factors—your potential and talent, educational preparation, deliberate practice, hard work, seeing and seizing opportunities, and being mentored.
- Becoming an expert nurse requires talent, time, and a team.
- Get to know your passions and talents and make them "reality" with the "you" and "other" factors.

RAISE YOUR MENTOR INTELLIGENCE FOR SUCCESS

You can increase your Mentor Intelligence by thoughtful planning and involvement in each of the three competencies of mentoring intelligence. This will prove to be a major step in your development as a professional nurse. First, a **mentoring mentality** means that you study the concept of mentoring and its benefits to you, your patients, and your profession. It is essential that you become knowledgeable about the mentoring process and how you can give and receive its benefits. Second, a **mentoring lens** means that you regard your colleagues, students, and yourself as needing and deserving mentoring assistance. You realize that every student and every nurse can benefit from receiving and giving mentoring, and that mentorship is a special investment in your colleagues' future success. You will reflect on how you can attract mentoring guidance to assist in the unfolding of your gifts. Further, you will make plans to be a mentor to specific students and colleagues as you gain strength and knowledge. The third aspect, **mentoring momentum**, means that you "live the mentor connection" in your relationships with other nurses and friends—that mentoring becomes a personal lifestyle as you share and learn with others.

=== *FAST FACTS in a NUTSHELL*

- You can raise your Mentor Intelligence by activating your mentoring mentality, your mentoring lens, and your mentoring momentum. Practice makes perfect. Practice everyday.
- Consciously choose to be an involved and committed mentor to students and colleagues as you grow professionally.

ONE-MINUTE MENTORING

A lot can happen in 60 seconds. In one minute someone can be helped or hurt by our supportive or negative messages. Our body language rapidly conveys either a mentoring "uplift" or "put down." One minute can provide a golden opportunity to mentor a student or colleague, or it can be a lost connection. You can ask a question and learn something new, or lose the moment. In one minute, you can show someone how to do a safe procedure, or not. One minute can be an enormously important mentoring event. **The bottom line: One minute is a precious opportunity for instant mentoring—an encouraging word, acknowledgment of a job well done, a teaching–learning moment, or networking with someone new.**

One-minute mentoring requires having a mentoring lens—a component of your Mentor Intelligence. This means that you are on the lookout for those moments when you notice a colleague or student in need of information, support, and encouragement; and you give it. Or you need some help, and you ask for it. You can create mentoring moments anywhere—in the classroom, on a nursing unit, at a meeting or a social event. One-minute mentoring is fast and efficient, gets quickly to the heart of the matter, and it works. In one minute you can give and receive the enormous benefits of mentoring. In one minute you can establish a valuable mentoring network for yourself. In one minute you can move another giant step up the ladder to professional success. **Each of us can be a one-minute mentor.**

BE THE "PERFECT" PROTÉGÉ

Since mentors are attracted to potential protégés whom they are willing to promote, it is important to know what the "attraction" factors are for mentors. As a protégé, leaving this to chance, or "catch-as-catch-can," is not a strategic way to attract mentoring. Since mentoring occurs between two people, there are many interpersonal considerations that affect "attraction." These include mutually shared values, interests, and goals; personal characteristics; talent; and "chemistry." Sometimes, opposites also attract. Mentors are particularly interested in potential, curiosity, eagerness to learn, and commitment. Leaders are always looking for the next generation of leaders—the "best and brightest" who will carry forth their legacy. There is no one-size-fits-all situation as to "attraction." Rather, a productive mentor–protégé relationship is dynamic and complementary and just seems to "fit."

Two studies conducted about the mentor–protégé relationship found three identical characteristics of the "ideal" protégé: intelligence, ambition, and willingness to take risks (Ensher & Murphy, 2005; Zey, 1984). These two studies, 20 years apart, differed on seven other qualities, however, which is probably due to changing times and the climate that shape mentors' ideas of the "perfect" protégé. The most recent study provides a comprehensive list of desirable qualities of the protégé (Ensher & Murphy, 2005):

- Intelligence
- Ambition
- Willingness to learn and take risks
- Initiative
- Energy
- Trustworthiness
- Integrity
- Emotional intelligence
- Optimism
- Complementary skills

An important point about being a "perfect" protégé is this: Because you have been singled out by mentors who go out of their way to help you above and beyond their usual responsibilities, you need to perform beyond the usual expectations. Studying and working hard—going the extra mile—is part of being a "perfect" protégé. One nurse leader puts in this way: "Mentorship is 'extra' work on both sides. You must be prepared to accept demands and expectations that are different from those others may be experiencing. It is this extra investment of all persons that makes mentorship rewarding and worthwhile" (Salmon, 1998, p. 69).

A real-life "perfect" protégé says that she believes because mentors have invested in her, she cannot disappoint them at any cost. Because she has been singled out for mentoring help from many corners, she is driven to excel above the usual standards. As she puts it, she has made a "commitment of the mind" to achievement in her performance. Through diligence in her advanced studies and her work responsibilities she stands head and shoulders "above the crowd," and has been recognized as an exceptional young leader through her positions and awards.

═══════════════════════════════════*FAST FACTS in a NUTSHELL*

- Take the initiative to meet new people, especially potential mentors, in professional and social situations.

Continued

Continued

- Be a One-Minute Mentor and look for students and colleagues who need a quick dose of support and encouragement. Also be on the lookout for One-Minute Mentors for yourself.
- Be a "perfect" protégé and attract mentors by your passion, energy, and commitment to perform and excel at a high level of expectation.
- If mentors have invested in you, do not disappoint them by being an "average" nurse, but work at your highest potential.

MENTORING VERSUS "TORMENTING" BEHAVIORS

If you possess Mentor Intelligence, you will not accept or tolerate the opposite of mentoring behaviors for you, your colleagues, and students. These are "tormenting" behaviors, and include disrespectful, intimidating behaviors that students and nurses may experience in school or on the job. They are barriers to learning, communication, collegial trust, professional development, and personal achievement. "Tormenting" behaviors include incivility, lateral violence, hazing, put-downs, bullying, and queen-beeism. We hear the negative expression, "eating our young," which describes the uncaring behaviors that some nurses and other health professional display with other nurses and students.

Perhaps you have witnessed these subtle and not-so-subtle put-downs of colleagues—the antithesis of mentoring. The presence, tolerance, and indifference to these toxic behaviors have been widely documented in the nursing literature (Dyess & Sherman, 2009; Griffin, 2004; Pellico, Brewer, & Kovner, 2009; Thomas & Burk, 2009). One of my students described it this way: "As a junior student, I was assigned to a preceptor who treated me as a 'nuisance.' She dismissed a procedural question I asked her by rolling her eyes and saying to another nurse, 'Nursing students are just not like they used to be.' She ridiculed me in the presence of my patient and a family member for not completing a dressing change as fast as she thought I should. The family member told me not to take it to heart, and that I was doing a good job. I felt totally humiliated and defeated."

The Joint Commission (2008) states that "intimidating and disruptive behaviors" can foster medical errors, contribute to poor patient satisfaction and preventable adverse outcomes, increase the cost of care, and cause employees to leave the organization. The Commission has issued a Sentinel Event Alert on *Behaviors That Undermine A Culture of Safety* (www.jointcommission.orgSentinelEvents/SentinelEventAlert/sea_40.htm). They state that these unprofessional behaviors "stem from both individual and system factors, including stress, high emotion situations, fatigue, immaturity, defensiveness, and self-centeredness." Toxic interpersonal behaviors can also arise from psychological oppression, anger, jealousy, and power-and-control needs. Nurses work in highly bureaucratic systems in which they may feel disrespected, unsupported, and powerless—leading to angry and oppressive behaviors toward colleagues.

Intimidating behaviors are dangerous because they threaten patient safety and the psychological safety of health care professionals. They are dangerous because they prevent the creation of caring collegial environments—**a mentoring culture**—in which learning and professional development can flourish—where students and nurses can become confident, competent, high-performance clinical leaders who provide the highest quality, safe patient care. Non-mentoring behaviors damage teamwork, open communication, and confidence building.

Disrespectful collegial behaviors also violate the *Standards of Nursing Practice and Professional Performance* (ANA, 2004; 2010) and the spirit of *Nursing's Code of Ethics* (ANA, 2001). These behaviors, including lateral violence and intimidation, must be stopped through awareness, acknowledgment ("naming it"), exposure, and education. The Joint Commission's statement (2008) on intimidating and disruptive behaviors calls for zero tolerance of these behaviors. A *Leadership Standard* addressing these behaviors has been adopted by the Joint Commission, and is now effective for all accreditation programs. The ANA's *Leadership Standard* (2010) states that the registered nurse "mentors colleagues for the advancement of nursing practice, the profession, and quality health care" (p. 55).

The National Student Nurses' Association (NSNA) 2010 House of Delegates approved a resolution to "support policy development and increased funding for research on lateral violence in nursing and to educate its constituents" about this issue (NSNA, 2010). At their 2001 and 2006 conventions, NSNA delegates also called for increased education and awareness to prevent workplace violence and the establishment of a professional workplace culture (NSNA, 2001, 2006).

Two approaches are recommended for nurses and students in order to reduce "tormenting" behaviors: (1) role modeling a counterculture of mentorship, learning, and development—in contrast to a work culture of "shame and blame"; and (2) adopting a zero tolerance of unprofessional, disruptive behaviors by bonding with caring colleagues, teachers, and administrators. Nurses are strong role models of caring for their patients. Nurses can be, and usually are, caring colleagues and mentors for each other. All nurses must be vigilant in addressing toxic behaviors and promote mentoring behaviors among nursing colleagues and nursing students. **Choose, by your example and behavior, to be a model of mentoring behaviors with colleagues in school and the clinical workplace.**

Each of us is capable of assisting in the creation of "places of realized potential" wherever we live and work (De Pree, 1997). These places can be a nursing unit, a nursing program, or a professional association. Such places relentlessly support people to realize their potential and to develop their unique talents. These are environments that give people opportunities to learn and grow—where mentoring and coaching thrive—where achievement and excellence are celebrated and mentors are applauded. A "tormenting" organization is a tragedy.

A mentoring organization is a gift. A mentoring organization provides each employee the opportunity to experience the incredible benefits and rewards of mentoring. Developing the expert performance of every student and every nurse on the health care team has enormous implications for quality, safe, and compassionate patient care. Realizing potential through mentoring cultures will produce nursing leaders who can reform patient care, clinical work environments, and the health care system. A culture of mentoring, as a "place of realized potential," is described in Exhibit 5.1.

Exhibit 5.1   Places of Realized Potential
(Max De Pree, 1997)

- A place of realized potential opens itself to change, to contrary opinion, to mystery of potential, to involvement, to unsettling ideas.
- Places of realized potential offer people opportunities to learn and grow.
- A place of realized potential offers the gift of challenging work.
- A place of realized potential sheds its obsolete baggage.
- A place of realized potential encourages people to decide what needs to be measured and then helps them do the work.

Continued

Exhibit 5.1 *Continued*

- A place of realized potential heals people with trust, caring, and with forgetfulness.
- People in places of realized potential know that organizations are social environments.
- A place of realized potential celebrates.

FAST FACTS in a NUTSHELL

- Do not accept intimidating "tormenting behaviors" directed to you, students, and colleagues.
- Disrespectful collegial behaviors can be stopped by awareness, acknowledgment, exposure, and education.
- Help to create "places of realized potential"— a mentoring culture—where sharing the gift of learning and mentoring with students, nurses, and other colleagues is valued and expected.
- Be a caring mentor to students and colleagues, and find the joy and satisfaction of seeing others reach their potential.

Making the "Mentor Match"

6

Networking: An Essential Mentoring Tool

We never know how our small activities will affect others through the invisible fabric of our connectedness. I have learned that in this exquisitely connected world, it's never a question of "critical mass." It's always about *crucial connections*. None of us exists independent of our relationships with others. . . . In each of these relationships, we are different, new in some way.

—Margaret Wheatley (1999)

INTRODUCTION

Networking is a cornerstone to your career success. Are you "connected?" Do you "connect" regularly with people in professional and social situations? Connecting with other people is what networking is all about. Networking is simply establishing relationships and connections with people. It is how people meet, get things done, exchange information and support, and find resources—including mentors. In essence, human networks make things happen. Networks are a function of what you know, who you know, and who you are. Becoming knowledgeable about the art and skills of networking, both face-to-face and electronic, is the focus of this chapter.

In this chapter, you will learn:

1. The basics of networks and networking
2. How and where to make connections
3. The successful networker's important skills and tools

THE NETWORK AND NETWORKING

A network is a web of interpersonal and technological connections and relationships. It includes all the linkages we have with each other—in our family, work, professional, and social life. Everyone needs to be well connected with people—it is how we're wired as human beings. It is how we interact and carry out our daily lives. It has been pointed out that "we don't just live in groups—we live in networks or webs of interactions that are repeated or sustained over time" (Christakis & Fowler, 2009).

Networking is establishing relationships and connections with others. We all need each other for information, assistance, advice, support, feedback, contacts, and affirmation. Networking makes all of these things happen. There are literally thousands of different types of networks that exist for different reasons. In the nursing profession, for example, there are numerous specialty associations that are highly organized to help their members connect face-to-face with each other. These networking connections serve many purposes: learning about new trends, skill development, information sharing through meetings and conferences, engaging in policy and political action, and of course, mentoring each other. It is essential that you become a member of these powerful nursing networks in order to gain access to valuable information and contacts.

In addition to our face-to-face networks, we increasingly rely on electronic connections—online social networks. Tapping into online networks, such as forums, discussion boards, listserve groups, and blogging sites, has become essential for expanding personal and professional contacts. Online social and professional engagement has created effective networking opportunities. Global sharing and electronic mentoring are now possible with professional colleagues around the world. Online social networking offers these advantages:

- Expands access to information
- Connects people with similar interests
- Provides a springboard for face-to-face networks

Remember that electronic networks do not replace traditional face-to-face networking. Instead, these electronic networks complement and increase opportunities for face-to-face networking. **The bottom line: The ideal** networking model capitalizes on both human and electronic contacts. Combining these two powerful modes of networking is the formula for success.

YOUR NETWORK TO SUCCESS

Do not take it lightly: Your individual network is essential to your career success. Therefore, careful thought, time, and energy should be spent in strategically cultivating your professional relationships. Networking is the "way in" to success. In order to be well connected to information, resources, and support, you need to seize opportunities to meet people and have them get to know **you**. An important way to discover mentors and have them discover **you** is through a variety of networking avenues.

It is a fact that the majority of positions in all fields are filled through networks of colleagues, friends, and Internet job sites. **Getting in the door** happens through information from human and Internet contacts—**what** you know. **Getting the job** happens through the human connection—**who** you know and **who** you are. Of two equally prepared candidates for a position, one will have the greater advantage if a personal connection is made on her/his behalf. Fair or not, it's how things work.

You described the composition of your network in the **Inventory of Mentor Networks** (Chapter 4, Exhibit 4.1). You can now use this inventory as a basis for deciding how to: (1) strengthen connections with people and groups **already** in your network; and (2) build **new** relationships with people and groups. The quality of these networks is more important than sheer quantity. For example, it is helpful to network with people who are "well connected," since they can open the doors to their extensive networks that will in turn increase your chances of meeting other well-connected people.

Your network should include nurses, other professionals, and people in your social, community, and family circles. It is very helpful to have a **variety** of good contacts. It is best if your networking connections cross many boundaries. This happens through having a variety of life roles. You may be a nurse, parent, community volunteer, member of professional associations, friend, health club member, graduate student, and so on. All of these roles and the activities associated with them offer you exciting networking opportunities.

What Networking Is Not

Networking is not "instant gratification." It takes an investment of personal time, attention, and patience to develop positive networks.

Networking is not just a "means to an end." Networking is a growth opportunity that can be as important as the outcome.

Networking is not a "one-way street." It is about sharing and giving to others, as well as receiving. The focus of networking should be on learning.

FAST FACTS in a NUTSHELL

- Networking is the process of establishing relationships and connections with people in order to "make things happen."
- Networks are a function of *what* you know, *who* you know, and *who* you are.
- Face-to-face and online social networking modes complement each other.
- Networking is not instantaneous, a means to an end, or a one-way street. Generosity is the key to positive networking.
- Networking is a cornerstone of your career success.

MAKING CONNECTIONS—HOW AND WHERE

Networking occurs everywhere and everyday—we all network daily. We just need to do it more consciously and with greater awareness and skill, so that it becomes a "way of thinking and being." Anytime that you are in contact with people is an opportunity to make connections. Dozens of these opportunities arise everyday in trains, stores, schools, gyms, hospitals, libraries, meetings—wherever people mix and mingle. Do not be shy. Practice your "people" skills. Get out there and consciously network. Strike up a conversation with someone while you're waiting in line, shopping, sitting on a bus, or in a coffee shop. People are out there to meet and connect with you.

The power of your network will depend on the variety of your interests, energy, and drive to get connected with the "right" people. An honest appraisal of your current network will be helpful. Carefully examine your **Inventory of Mentor Networks** to determine both strengths and gaps in your network. This audit will provide valuable clues about what you need to do to get better connected. Remember that our networks are always a dynamic work-in-progress.

Increasing your knowledge about networking from various sources will be helpful as you build your network. You will find numerous books, articles, seminars, and Internet resources that discuss networking and how to do it. The best approach is to just jump in—and **practice, practice, practice**. Being a member of the nursing profession is a great advantage for networking. As nurses we all have had the experience of introducing ourselves as a nurse at a social event or meeting, and we immediately become the focus for many questions and conversation. **Nurses have a strong networking advantage for sharing and making connections.**

BE A RELENTLESS NETWORKER

Since networking is the way to make things happen, being an active networker will make positive things happen in your career. This means that you reach out constantly—daily—to other people. Although you don't always realize it, you network all the time. The key to your success is being more **aware** and **strategic** about it.

Tap into Multiple Networks

There are endless networking sources—informal and formal. Cast your "net" widely. Every group, work organization, or association that you belong to is an excellent networking source for learning, making new contacts, and sharing information. These groups have Web sites and special networking events for the express purpose of helping people meet and share ideas. These events are fun and educational. It is not unusual to meet someone who inspires, entertains, or teaches you something.

- **Activate your Mentor Network Inventory.** Nurture and thank those individuals and groups already in your network for all they do for you. Make a plan to contact individuals or join groups that you have identified as potentially useful to you. Then do it—no procrastination.
- **Network through groups and organizations.** These include professional associations, which are extensive in the nursing and health care fields. Other promising opportunities are workplace committees, alumni associations, volunteer groups, colleges, community and school boards, political clubs, workshops, and conferences. Some groups have developed an online Community of Mentors to share information and help each other with various issues.
- **Look for online social networking opportunities.** Search for online business and professional networking sites. Online networking platforms include Facebook, Twitter, LinkedIn.com, Meetup.com, Google groups,

blogs, listserve groups, and Monster.com. Nursing online networks include the professional association Web sites that may have threaded forums, discussion boards, and information available to members only. For additional ideas, see **Appendix B: Resources for Collective Mentoring and Networking**.

- **Be strategic. Set goals.**
  - ○ Attend at least one meeting or event every month.
  - ○ Try to meet someone new every week.
  - ○ Check out a new Internet site.
  - ○ Network through various online platforms.
  - ○ Invite someone to lunch or coffee.
  - ○ Make an appointment with a potential mentor.
  - ○ Read a book or article and share ideas with someone.
  - ○ Volunteer to be a mentor to children, young people, and students.
  - ○ Ask someone to work with you on a special project.
  - ○ Take a course at a museum, college, or community organization.
  - ○ Volunteer at a political or community event.

═══════════════════════*FAST FACTS in a NUTSHELL*

- Networking should be a daily event—make it work for you.
- Nurture your *current* network, and add *new* individuals and groups.

Continued

Continued

- Network widely with individuals, organizations, associations—in person and online.
- Be strategic and creative in finding and expanding your networks and mentors.
- Remember that your network should always be changing and growing.

TAKE ACTION FOR SUCCESS

It can't be emphasized enough—you must make a positive impression in your networking encounters.

> Networking is a contact sport. You get exactly one chance to make that all-important first impression. People who are meeting you for the first time are judging you, whether you want them to or not...and this "sizing up" is done in seven seconds (Misner, 2008).

Whether we realize it or not, in a few seconds, we tend to judge someone from an initial interaction in a networking situation and form a quick perception of that person and that perception becomes reality for us.

Be **professional** in your self-presentation. Your overall appearance, body language, dress, manners, speech, and engagement with others all play a role in whether your networking works for or against you. Take a look in the mirror and determine what visual message you send as you interact with people. **Caution:** Be aware of the impact of the following items, particularly in light of how different generations of nurses and other health care professionals might view them: tattoos, body piercings, nails, hair styles and coloring, flip flops and sandals, cut of shirts and skirts, and iPod usage.

It is believed that 80%–90% of communication power comes from nonverbal cues, such as body language. The quality of your handshake, eye contact, posture, attire, and mannerisms are a photographic message in your encounter, and leave an impression—for better or worse. Be friendly and genuinely interested in others. Be a good listener. Offer to help others when you can. Giving to others in networking encounters is the key, not getting or taking. The rewards come from generosity in the process and the ripple effects of that sharing.

Check out your communication skills. Choice of words and voice quality and pitch are significant factors. Your speaking, telephone, and electronic skills, and written messages are powerful representations of you, so refine them. Do you speak clearly, concisely, and with confidence? E-mail addresses and e-messages are an area for careful assessment. **Caution:** Is your electronic address "professional," seductive, or "silly"? Are your telephone messages so brief and informal that they border on being rude and impossible to understand? Does your Facebook, blog, or Twitter contain information that you would not want potential employers or professional colleagues to see?

Get feedback from trusted friends and colleagues about your personal presentation and their suggestions for improvement. Openness to learning, self-awareness, and self-correction will make the difference between being a poor, average, or superb (successful) networker. Remember that a big aspect of networking is **self-marketing**. Exquisite networking is required if you want to be a serious professional nurse with a serious professional career.

NETWORKING TOOLS

These include an up-to-date resume, business cards, address books (print and electronic), and electronic networking sites.

- **Resume:** Your resume is a statement of your personal and professional background and should reflect the best marketing statement about you and your accomplishments. It is your entrée to getting in the door for professional interviews, memberships, awards, scholarships, and other professional opportunities. While you develop, draft, and proofread your resume, ask your colleagues, teachers, and mentors for their suggestions. The careful time you invest in creating an exceptional "perfect" resume will yield excellent returns. The cover letter accompanying your resume should also be "perfect," with correct grammar, punctuation, and a professional "tone." Both the resume and cover letter should be printed on high quality, white- or buff-colored paper. No "bells and whistles"—just "plain professional."

- **Business Cards:** Every professional needs a business card to be a good networker. Business cards are a way to introduce yourself and to cement face-to-face professional and/or social contacts. Cards may be provided by your employer. If not, get your own cards made at a print store or the Internet (e.g., VistaPrint.com). Your business card should be simple and straightforward—no fancy designs. When you get your business cards, have them with you **at all times.** Carry them in a card case or in your wallet, particularly when you attend social and professional events. You never know whom you might meet or what networking contact may arise. To be caught without this networking tool is a lost opportunity. **Note:** Electronic sites are increasingly the new wave of exchanging professional contacts. The same professional approach holds.

- **Address Books:** Whether they are electronic or on paper, your contact lists are crucial for ongoing referrals, sharing information, and strengthening and expanding your contacts. Various electronic network sites provide opportunities for storing your professional background and information, and for networking with people in nursing and other professions.

FAST FACTS in a NUTSHELL

- Capitalize on both face-to-face and electronic networking opportunities.
- A positive and professional presentation of yourself is essential for networking success.
- Maintain up-to-date professional networking tools, including your resume, business cards, address books, and electronic sites.

7

Negotiating the
Mentor–Protégé "Match"

Mentoring is a song of power that becomes embedded in the very fabric of one's existence. When in doubt, nurses must sing the song of mentoring—the song of hope, power, and direction.... The song of mentoring needs to shake and shape the walls of the nursing profession to generate leaders....

—Beverly Malone (1998)

INTRODUCTION

Your mentor intelligence will help bring mentors into your life. Attracting and keeping good mentors is a major developmental task in your career, beginning in the early years and throughout your professional life. Establishing a productive mentoring relationship requires a positive attitude and some ground rules. The mentor–protégé relationship changes over time, and each distinct phase provides opportunities and challenges for growth and learning. Mentors are transitional figures who come into your life and guide you at important career points.

In this chapter, you will learn:

1. How to find and keep mentors
2. Compatibilities that contribute to the mentoring "match"
3. Ground rules for productive mentoring
4. Transitions in the mentor–protégé relationship

GETTING STARTED: CHOICE AND EXPECTATIONS

Becoming familiar with the enormous advantages of having mentors in your life and career will be a great motivator to search for them. Once you establish your career goals and interests, you can then determine what you are looking for in your mentors, and what you want to gain in a mentoring relationship. You might be "chosen" by mentors, and you can also be the "chooser." In addition, you can be "matched" with mentors in a formal organizational program.

Choose Mentors Widely and Wisely

We know that **mentors are everywhere**—look for them wherever you are. Active networking—casting a wide net—is imperative for finding mentors. As discussed in Chapter 4, there are two approaches to finding mentors who can work for you in your career growth and development.

- A **free choice**, or choosing your own mentors, happens spontaneously and informally—the way most relationships begin. Mentors and protégés frequently choose each other this way.
- An **arranged match** occurs in formal mentor programs that are offered to employees in the workplace, to students in nursing programs, and to members of professional associations.

You will also wisely have both **expert** and **peer mentors** in your repertoire of support relationships. The more, the merrier! Nurses find that they benefit from both kinds of mentors, particularly at transitional points throughout their career. Since professional development lasts a lifetime, you will have many opportunities to share with and learn from different kinds of mentors.

- **Expert mentors** are more advanced in their career and can offer you the benefit of their experience and wisdom and open many doors to guidance, networking, ideas, opportunities, information, and people. These mentors can ask you important questions and help you to see the big picture in your career.
- **Peer mentors** are in your "league," so to speak; and each of you can share experiences, learn together, and give each other feedback and support.

Clarify Expectations

A careful examination of your career goals and mentoring expectations will guide you in finding the right "match." This is the first step. Take stock of yourself—your values, goals, strengths, needs, and interests. Be honest about whether you are ready and willing to invest your time and energy in a goal-directed support relationship. Openness and a curiosity to learn are crucial qualities in a mentor relationship.

Review again the **Mentor Readiness Assessment** (Chapter 3, Exhibit 3.1). This assessment will help clarify your goals and expectations about mentoring. In addition, the following questions will highlight some specific aspects about what you think would help you in a mentor relationship. Feedback and discussion with your peers in a class or with colleagues is recommended.

- What are my dreams and goals?
- What specific talents and skills do I want to develop?
- In what ways do I think mentoring could help me reach my dreams and goals?
- What would my "ideal" mentor look like? What should I realistically expect from a mentor relationship?
- What qualities of a potential mentor would "fit" with me and my specific values, aspirations, and needs?
- How much am I willing to invest in this mentor relationship?

In the early stages of a mentoring relationship, a frank and explicit discussion about the responsibilities and expected benefits for each person should occur. Each person brings different experiences, motives, and emotions to a relationship—this is also true in mentoring relationships. Both mentors and protégés should discuss their expectations as openly and honestly as possible and agree on mutually acceptable approaches to these expectations. Taking time early in the relationship for this discussion will go a long way in preventing misunderstanding and disappointments.

FAST FACTS in a NUTSHELL

- Mentors and protégés find each other by "choice" and/or by an arranged "match."
- Both expert and peer mentors are invaluable resources and provide different benefits.
- Expectations are a big influence on the quality and outcomes of mentor relationships and should be openly discussed and clarified.

ATTRACTORS AND COMPATIBILITIES: DO WE MATCH?

An emotional connection and/or respect are "**attractors**" in the early stages of a mentor relationship. Studies have shown that **similarity** of various attributes of the mentor and protégé contributes to a compatible relationship and successful outcomes. These include similarities of career goals, personality traits, personal and professional values, communication skills, and career commitment.

Mentors are particularly attracted to potential protégés by such qualities as a strong work ethic, drive, ambition, and enthusiasm. Some mentors claim they choose protégés who remind them of themselves and their aspirations and dreams. Some mentors choose protégés who aspire to be nurses with similar professional values, goals, and attitudes. In turn, protégés are attracted to mentors who are successful, inspirational, generous, and trustworthy. Protégés are also drawn to mentors whom they admire as role models and would like to emulate. Protégés should look for mentors who are respectful and interested in them and who are willing to invest time and energy on behalf of their goals.

It is important to note that **diversity** of age, gender, race, culture, ethnicity, and religion are not barriers to establishing productive mentoring relationships. Indeed, differences in characteristics and backgrounds among mentoring partners can generate innovative ideas, creative learning opportunities, and new perspectives. Professional partnerships that tap into "differences" offer a wealth of experiences and understanding that can enrich our careers and lives in many ways. "... Mentoring is a two-way street: intergenerational, transcultural, boundless" (Sinetar, 1998, p. 131).

====*FAST FACTS in a NUTSHELL*

- "Attractors" are qualities that draw mentors and protégés together, and include shared values and goals, work ethic, achievement needs, passion, and career commitment.

Continued

Continued

• Both similarities and differences in the personal attributes of mentors and protégés can contribute to innovative, transformative patterns of working and living.

WORKING TOGETHER: SOME GROUND RULES

Whether the mentor–protégé relationship is chosen or is arranged, or the mentor is an expert or a peer, establishing some ground rules for working together will promote a productive relationship. The basic ingredients for a successful, satisfying mentoring relationship are the same as for any other relationship—mutual trust, respect, interest, and open communication. Confidence and belief in each other will build a mutual commitment to the relationship. In the early stages of the relationship, the mentoring partners should discuss and mutually agree on: (1) goals and expectations, (2) time management, (3) work approaches and boundaries, and (4) feedback opportunities.

Goals and Expectations

In the beginning, it is very important to have candid conversations about what the protégé hopes to achieve career-wise, as well as the information and support that the mentor can realistically provide. This provides clarity and focus for meetings and for "measuring" success. The discussion should include: What do we want to accomplish? How will we know if we achieved our objectives? What are our responsibilities as protégé and as mentor for moving forward the "goal agenda"? What can each of us bring to the "success equation?"

A written working plan that is developed by the protégé and shared with the mentor will provide focus. This plan is a work-in-progress, of course, as it will change in response to the dynamic nature of working together. As goals are achieved, the protégé and mentor will undoubtedly discover new information and different challenges. A working plan can include the following: (1) the protégé's needs, goals, and expectations; (2) approaches and time lines; and (3) review of key results.

Time Management

Mentors are busy people; they can't afford to waste time and effort. The working plan described earlier will provide structure for mentoring interactions and promote efficiency of time and effort. General ground rules for time management may include frequency and context of contacts, best ways to contact each other (telephone, e-mail, texting), careful preparation for meetings, and prompt follow-up of plans. Time "drifting" is a common problem in busy people's relationships and can be avoided by developing some implicit and explicit ground rules.

Work Approaches and Boundaries

How mentors and protégés work together is a very personal matter. To prevent misunderstanding and promote healthy interactions, relationship boundaries should be reviewed. Sometimes mentors and protégés have multiple roles with each other that overlap and bring them together in varied settings, such as classes, meetings, social gatherings, and travel. To avoid inappropriate violation of personal boundaries, some working assumptions should be negotiated. These include the following:

- Roles and responsibilities of the protégé and mentor
- Availability, work ethic, and working style of the mentoring partners
- Expectations and protocols for confidentiality
- Communication: Is it two way, honest, and direct?
- Conflict: Is it acknowledged and managed positively?

Feedback Opportunities

A mentor is an "honest mirror." Asking mentors for feedback is an invitation for them to share their views about you and your performance. Asking for feedback requires trust, humility, and openness. It indicates a keen desire to improve, and is a powerful way for you to learn and grow. Mentors have a unique perspective to give honest, helpful feedback to their protégés and to ask tough questions. Your mentors are on your side; they want you to shine; and they can offer invaluable advice and guidance for staying on the right track. The mutual exchange of feedback between honest and respectful mentoring partners provides excellent reciprocal learning opportunities.

Protégés should regularly ask for feedback. Not seeking feedback from your mentors is missing a great opportunity. Asking for feedback does not require you, the protégé, to blindly accept observations and suggestions. You should consider the advice of mentors, but ultimately you have to make your decisions. Feedback data are one of several tools for self-reflection and self-improvement.

A feedback model to guide feedback communication between mentors and protégés was developed by Zachary (2005, 2009). This model suggests that protégés **ask** for feedback, **receive** feedback, **accept** feedback, **act** on feedback, and **give** feedback. These behaviors indicate your ownership, responsibility, and action for feedback. The continuous nature of this feedback cycle will encourage you and your mentor to engage in feedback at any point in the cycle. **The bottom line: "Success in meeting your goals and getting the most out of your mentoring relationships depends on your ability to draw on the feedback you get from your mentor (and others) and to act on it effectively"** (Zachary, 2009, p. 92).

════════════════════════════*FAST FACTS in a NUTSHELL*

- The basic ingredients of a productive, fulfilling mentoring relationship include reciprocal trust, respect, interest, and open communication.

Continued

Continued

- Important ground rules for working together include mutual understanding about goals and expectations, time management, work approaches and boundaries, and feedback opportunities.

TRANSITIONS IN THE RELATIONSHIP

Because of its human nature, mentoring relationships are developmental and transitional. They begin, change, mature, evolve, and perhaps end. A mentor relationship may consist of a "mentoring moment," or may last for years or decades. There is **generational mentoring**, in which mentors "grow" mentors who "grow" other mentors in a legacy effect, like a pebble thrown in a stream. Research has shown that on average, traditional mentor relationships last eight years, but this is highly variable. Many mentoring relationships in the nursing profession have been known to exist for decades as they change and evolve in an expanding circle of sharing and involvement. Mentors and protégés often continue to influence each other beyond original expectations—very much like the teacher–student and parent–child relationship. People are changed forever by human relationships. The mentor relationship is one of those life-changing connections.

Regardless of the duration, there are several developmental stages in the mentor relationship (Johnson & Ridley, 2004). These are approximate guides and may not apply to every relationship. The **beginning or initiation** phase starts with getting to know each other and establishing ground rules for the relationship. The **cultivation or working** phase is the active, intensive work period, in which the mentoring partners collaborate in both career and personal activities. The **separation** phase entails substantial structural, time, psychological, or developmental changes in the relationship. In the **redefinition or evolving** phase, the relationship evolves into a different, less intense form; but the relationship still exists through mutual respect, inspiration, and advocacy.

Transitions and developmental changes are inherent in mentoring relationships. There are bound to be feelings of loss for the partners as the relationship becomes less intense. At the same time, a deep sense of pride and gratitude for what was shared provides an enormous feeling of satisfaction. This is very much like the growth transition of children "leaving the nest" of the parents and flying on their own. This means success. As one mentor put it:

> I have to recognize from the beginning that she [my protégé] might, and in all probability will, exceed me in both educational and professional accomplishments. It is important that I take this as a compliment to my tutelage and not as a threat to my importance (J. Brucker, 1998).

Review and Evaluation

From the beginning of the mentor relationship through each evolving phase, it is essential to engage in ongoing review and evaluation of the protégé's changing needs, career goals, personal expectations, and key outcomes. This review provides data to help the mentoring partners change the focus, form, or direction of the relationship, as indicated. It is an excellent opportunity for the protégé to engage in self-reflection and career analysis and to give and receive honest feedback with the mentor. Evaluation is central to the learning process in mentor relationships. Review and evaluation help both mentor and protégé to gain insight and confidence to move forward with new challenges and new goals. Reciprocal rewards are always part of mentoring outcomes.

FAST FACTS in a NUTSHELL

- Mentor relationships are characterized by transitional, developmental stages with distinct characteristics.
- Ongoing review and evaluation of the mentor relations will help determine if the protégé's needs and goals are being well served.
- Mentors and protégés have a powerful influence on each other throughout their lives and careers, although the degree and frequency of the relationship changes.

8

Troubleshooting the Mentor Relationship

The mentor is not obligated to you for life. Nor are you obligated to be a protégé for life. You are obligated, however, to be respectful of each other, to recognize each other for the time you spent together...and be thankful for the pearls of wisdom you received.

—Wickman and Sjodin (1997)

INTRODUCTION

The mentor relationship, because it is human, is not perfect. As with all relationships, misunderstandings and conflicts may emerge. The enormous benefits to both the mentor and the protégé far outweigh any difficulties, but you should be aware of relational challenges. Being an informed participant can help you make the most of mentoring, through awareness of potential problems and the management of any difficulties.

In this chapter, you will learn:

1. The importance of risk prevention in mentor relationships
2. About potential roadblocks for mentors and protégés
3. How to manage change in the mentoring experience

RISK PREVENTION: BE INFORMED

Mentor relationships are an invaluable component in a nurse's career and should be entered into with thought and care. These relationships are special; there is nothing quite like them in one's life and work. They require commitment of time and involvement on the part of both mentors and protégés to achieve worthwhile results. Therefore, you should fully understand the nature of mentoring so that disappointments can be avoided.

> Mentorships are similar to other relationships in one important respect: they are imperfect and subject to human foibles. Some mentorships become riddled by conflict, dissatisfaction, or result in difficult endings. Some become unhealthy and dysfunctional (Johnson & Ridley, 2004).

Awareness of potential problems is important. Being informed about choosing "good" mentors, what is required to make the collaboration worthwhile, and how to negotiate the relationship are key to preventing problems.

Know what assumptions and expectations are held by you and your mentors. Problems can occur due to inadequate information, misunderstanding, and unclear expectations about the collaboration. For example, having unrealistically high expectations about the protégé's goals may lead to disillusionment for both mentoring partners. Through candid, honest conversations, decisions about mutually agreed upon expectations can be reached. Being "on the same page" is the best guarantee for productive goal-oriented work and for avoiding disillusionment.

Ask yourself if your expectations of your mentoring relationships are realistic and reasonable. Are you and your mentor(s) in agreement with your goals and expectations? Do you expect miracles or support from mentoring? Good risk prevention includes agreeing with your mentors on basic expectations about your goals and outcomes, frequency of contact, roles your mentor can play, expected performance of both partners, and how to address problems if they arise.

As the relationship develops, each person should respect the personal boundaries of each other. Regular feedback and honest communication are proven approaches to prevent misunderstanding and for problem solving.

═══════════════════════════════*FAST FACTS in a NUTSHELL*

- Enter the mentor relationship with awareness of limitations and challenges.
- Realistic expectations and a good "match" of personal and professional characteristics help prevent relationship derailment.
- Mutual feedback and honest communication are at the heart of healthy mentoring.

CAUTION: ROADBLOCKS

Although the majority of mentoring relationships are positive and productive, some difficulties can arise. These stem from the pressures of work and daily life, time demands, or personal issues. Studies have reported various types of mentoring relationship problems such as: (1) unrealistic expectations, (2) personal and professional mismatches, (3) power and control issues, (4) excessive competitiveness, (5) "cloning," (6) communication, and (7) dependence (Vance & Olson, 1998).

Unrealistic expectations. Mentors and protégés bring high hopes to the mentoring relationship. These can be realistic expectations—or they can be too low, too high, or inappropriate. As a result, if the expectations are not met, disappointment and feelings of betrayal can appear. Mentoring is not a panacea for success in attaining every professional goal. Make sure you have realistic expectations about the contributions that mentoring can contribute to your career, and discuss these candidly with your mentors.

Personal and professional mismatches. Respect and "chemistry" attract mentors and protégés to each other and enhance the growth of the relationship. There should be some basic similarities of personality qualities and professional values, or the relationship may hit roadblocks. Differences also can enrich the quality of learning in the relationship. At the same time, a strong "mutual match" of qualities is helpful for bonding with each other and committing to the protégé's goals. Some of these include similar values, career commitment, work style, and communication approaches.

Power and control issues. A power differential usually exists between protégés and mentors, particularly in expert-to-novice mentoring; and this differential should be acknowledged. Mentors have enormous influence with their protégés due to their power of knowledge, reputation, expertise, wisdom, and affirmation. Power and shared power (empowerment) should always be employed to enhance the talent and potential of the protégé. Abuses of power in the mentor relationship occur when there are instances of manipulation, exploitation, intimidation, and excessive demands of loyalty and conformity by the mentor.

Excessive competitiveness. A degree of competition among colleagues, including mentors and protégés, is normal and healthy. Excessive competitiveness, however, weakens trust and mutual sharing among protégés and their mentors. This, in turn, erodes opportunities for trust and sharing,

"Cloning." As a protégé, you should strive to reach **your** dreams and realize **your** unique potential. This is your goal! You should not try to be a carbon copy of anyone else. It is hazardous if mentors expect protégés to demonstrate excessive "likeness" of themselves. Imitation and modeling are positive aspects of mentoring, but should always be in the service of supporting the development of the protégé's unique qualities and talents.

Communication. Frequent, open, and honest communication is the foundation of healthy mentor relationships. Truth telling with compassion is the best approach. One of the mentor's gifts is serving as a sounding board—listening, reflecting, and giving feedback. Other gifts from the mentor are asking tough questions, playing the "devil's advocate," and presenting a landscape of options.

Dependence. Protégés should make their own independent decisions with input, guidance, and encouragement from mentors. Protégés must be proactive in the relationship and take the initiative as much as possible. It is **your** career, and no one else's! Having multiple mentors provides different perspectives and experiences. It is highly recommended that you establish a "board of mentors," consisting of both peer and expert members, who can offer you a variety of vantage points.

FAST FACTS in a NUTSHELL

- Relational roadblocks may potentially exist in mentoring relationships.
- There are usually "warning labels" that may alert mentoring partners to potential problems.
- Regular communication and feedback between the mentoring partners ensure success.
- Develop a "board of mentors" who can bring a diversity of perspectives and experiences to your career.

MANAGING CHANGE

Since the mentor relationship inevitably changes over time, there will be experiences that bring incredible joy and some that cause doubt and sadness. As with all human encounters, conflicts may arise, disappointments occur, and conflicting emotions will emerge.

Be realistic. Nothing is perfect, and mentoring is not a miracle solution to all career matters. Problems may arise over the life of the relationship. Planning for change at the very beginning of the relationship will diminish surprises and disillusionment. Stages in the changing mentor relationship will bring different challenges and conflicts—this is a normal sequence of events.

Acknowledge change and conflict. These should be faced head on. The mentor and protégé should have candid conversations about "issues" and attempt to resolve them. Positive problem solving works if the relationship is built on a foundation of mutual trust. Applying good conflict management skills is helpful. Conflict intervention, characterized by respect and honesty, can strengthen the relationship and promote the maturation of both mentoring partners.

Get feedback. "The most productive mentorships are those in which both parties actively participate in a systematic process of evaluation that aids in the protégé's professional development" (Johnson & Ridley, 2004, p. 83). It is imperative to keep an open attitude of inquiry about the process of the relationship and to "tweak" it to meet the goals of the relationship. Periodic discussions to determine whether the relationship is meeting the protégé's needs will guide decisions about maintaining, changing, or ending the relationship. Give-and-take feedback can address changing expectations, needs, and circumstances, and needs of the mentoring partners. **The bottom line: Regular feedback is a major contributor to managing changes in mentoring relationships.**

Redefinition or Separation in the Relationship

Like good parents, good mentors will help protégés "grow up" and fly on their own. There will come a time when the intensity and involvement of the relationship changes, just like the ever-changing relationship between parent–child and teacher–student. The best outcome is that protégés mature and are launched on their own path. This should not be seen as the diminishment of the mentor's influence, but rather as an enormous tribute to the mentor's skill and generosity. The relationship may live on, but in a changed form. Unfortunately, some relationships may end due to dysfunctional conflicts.

Mentors are transitional figures that come in and out of one's life. There will be normal feelings of loss when mentors and protégés redefine or separate from the relationship. Self-reflection and review of a positive mentoring relationship will most likely elicit various feelings of satisfaction, gratitude, joy, and sadness. The growth and achievements stemming from the mentor relationship are a reminder of the power and magic of mentoring. A true mentoring experience is filled with the riches of sharing, support, and the excitement of discovery. It is one of those mountaintop life experiences that make everything feel different!

=*FAST FACTS in a NUTSHELL*

- Be aware of and acknowledge change and conflict in the mentor relationship.
- Review and re-evaluate the relationship as it proceeds through various stages.
- The protégé's best interests must always be at the forefront in a mentoring relationship.
- Mentor relationships are transitional and may continue over a lifetime, or come to an end.
- The power and magic of mentor relationships are reflected in the achievements, joyful sharing, and professional and life connections between mentoring partners.

PART

IV

Career Success and the Mentor Connection

9

Passing the Torch of Success: Becoming a Mentor–Leader

Those who have torches will pass them to others.

—Plato

Each of us is capable of being a mentor in one way or another. If we think about leaving a legacy, we will establish these relationships, because mentoring is really a crucial element to growth. A million mentors wouldn't be too many!

—De Pree (1997)

INTRODUCTION

Each nurse at every career stage can become a mentor and a leader. The growth, success, and well-being of nurses and the nursing profession largely depend on nurses helping each other be the best nurses they can be. When nurses mentor, lead, and teach each other, everyone benefits—individual nurses, our patients, the nursing profession, and the clinical workplace. When nurses don't mentor each other, their ability to provide the highest quality nursing care is compromised. Since there are always people ahead and behind us in our development, we have limitless opportunities to help and be helped by each other. The multigenerational nature of nursing and the presence of workplace diversity also provide creative opportunities for mentoring, leading, and learning.

In this chapter, you will learn:

1. About becoming a mentor–leader: Beliefs and behaviors
2. Mentoring across cultures and generations
3. Mentor as Pygmalion: Believing in potential and expecting success

ARE YOU A LEADER?

Hopefully, every nurse believes that she/he is a leader. Nurses *are* leaders by virtue of their expertise and knowledge, the legal sanction of their work, their essential role in society, and the attributes they possess as professionals. Do you see yourself as a leader? Do you assume leadership functions in your nursing practice?

There are literally hundreds of definitions of leadership. However, a few key components are present in most definitions. We know, for example, that leaders: (1) influence others; (2) accomplish their work through cultivating relationships; and (3) develop others through teaching and mentoring. Theorists point out that there are three foci of leadership: people, things, and ideas—or the human, technical, and conceptual. The "people" aspect of leadership is considered the most significant because work is carried out with people. Having "people" skills (i.e., possessing emotional and social intelligence) is crucial to being an effective leader (Goleman, Boyatzis, & McKee, 2002). Empathy, compassion, and advocacy are some of the characteristics of the "people" leader. Nurses and nursing students epitomize these qualities as they serve others through their mission of caring and healing.

The "art" of leadership lies in liberating and polishing gifts of others (De Pree, 1989; 1992). The best leaders—and mentors—inspire others to believe in their potential and possibilities—to try new ways of being and working. Every novice and every expert nurse should be a mentor–leader. Leaders are not defined or limited by title, position, experience, age, gender, or sociocultural background. Leadership is a privileged position of serving others. It is crucial to **believe** you are a leader and to **behave** like a leader, even in the early stages of your career.

It is never too early to begin testing your leadership behaviors, especially under the tutelage of more experienced nurses and teachers as well as peer and expert mentors. Becoming a leader is a developmental learning process—it takes desire, time, and experience. You can learn leadership by: (1) observing good leaders, mentors, and role models; (2) studying leadership theories and research; (3) testing leadership behaviors through work and professional association activities; (4) seeking feedback from your mentors and colleagues; and

(5) using reflective learning to develop and fine-tune your behaviors. Writing regularly in a journal about your leadership experiences and discussing these with your mentors and colleagues is an excellent leadership learning experience.

BECOMING A MENTOR–LEADER

The qualities of good leaders and mentors are similar. Leadership and mentorship are concerned with the development and empowerment of others. Mentors, like leaders, help colleagues realize their potential and help them liberate their unique gifts. One protégé states: "I was going through the motions of my education, like 'sleepwalking' without seeing a picture of where I was headed, and who I could be. My mentors woke me up, and helped me see the big picture—that I could be a leader—and how to proceed to make it 'real.'" One study found that relationships with peers, mentors, and patients were directly instrumental in nurses' ability to perform at higher levels of expertise and leadership (Roche, Morsi, & Chandler, 2009).

BELIEFS AND BEHAVIORS OF THE MENTOR–LEADER

In order to become an effective mentor–leader, you will need to possess certain beliefs and exhibit professional behaviors. Beliefs are major determinants of behavior. If you believe you can be and/or are a leader, then your behaviors will reflect that belief system. Assess your beliefs and behaviors about your leadership and mentoring activities through the following Checklist. Your answers will provide clues about your intent and abilities to cultivate relationships as a mentor–leader.

A Checklist of Beliefs and Behaviors for Being a Mentor–Leader			
My Assessment Statements	*Yes*	*No*	*Not Sure*
Beliefs			
I see myself as a leader.			
I see myself as a mentor.			
Mentoring is an essential professional activity.			
Every nurse should have mentoring relationships with both peers and experts.			
I believe in my colleagues' potential and expect them to be successful.			
I believe that mentoring is both a privilege and an obligation.			

Continued

Continued			
My Assessment Statements	Yes	No	Not Sure
I value the contributions of diverse cultures and generations on the nursing team.			
Behaviors			
I actively mentor others.			
I actively seek mentors among my peers and expert colleagues.			
I am a role model for professional performance in collegiality, collaboration, and leadership.			
I exhibit professional behaviors in my communication, dress, demeanor, and relationships with my team.			
I am studying the concepts of leadership and mentorship.			
I have joined professional associations to gain experience in leadership and mentoring.			
I network daily in my contacts with colleagues and patients.			

═══════════════════════════ *FAST FACTS in a NUTSHELL*

- The professional nurse and nursing student have potential to become leaders by believing and behaving like a leader, in addition to preparation, motivation, and mentoring support.
- Mentors and leaders are visionaries who inspire and motivate others to realize their potential for success as leaders.
- The mentor–leader creates empowering, developmental relationships with students, peers, and expert colleagues.

MENTORING ACROSS CULTURES AND GENERATIONS

Mentor–leaders are present in every cultural and ethnic group and in every generation. Global, cross-cultural, and cross-generational mentoring occur when nurses are open and receptive to learning from each other and are willing to share their unique perspectives and skills. "The culture of nursing, with its value and perspective of caring, provides a framework of unity amidst diversity in mentoring" (Vance & Olson, 1998). The nursing profession has an impressive track record of global collaboration and mentorship. Through mentor bonds that break down global and cultural boundaries, nurses have unprecedented opportunities for driving change in health and nursing around the world.

Likewise, the different generations—the veterans, the baby boomers, the gen-Xers, and the millennials—with their different perspectives and values—can provide unique contributions that enhance the work of the entire health team. Differences can create misunderstandings and conflict, but the point is to recognize and value the differences by not stereotyping and judging. Generational cross-pollination and mentoring among the different generations can create excellent opportunities for creative problem solving, innovative approaches, excitement about learning, and the sheer fun of discovery.

===================*FAST FACTS in a NUTSHELL*

- Cultural and generational diversity can enliven mentor relationships through creativity and transformative approaches to learning and creative thinking.

MENTOR AS PYGMALION: BELIEVE IN POTENTIAL AND EXPECT SUCCESS

A Greek legend about a sculptor named Pygmalion adds another dimension to the mentor phenomenon. Pygmalion carved his "ideal" woman out of ivory and so deeply admired his sculpture that he prayed to Venus to make her come "alive." His belief and expectation about her and her virtues were rewarded; and she was transformed into a "real" woman, known as Galatea.

This engaging legend has been recreated in various art forms, including the Broadway play, "My Fair Lady." The core lesson of the Pygmalion story is that **one person's beliefs and expectations have a powerful, transformative effect on another person's behavior**. This effect acts as a kind of "self-fulfilling prophecy." In other words, what you expect is what you get! The mentoring phenomenon, like the Pygmalion concept, is a creator of human transformation.

You are indeed lucky if you can find Pygmalion–Mentors who **believe** in you and your potential, and who **expect** you to succeed in your career. If a protégé is viewed and treated as someone deserving of advocacy and special attention, the protégé will "buy into" the mentor's beliefs, and therefore **act** on that belief. It has been found that the mentor's belief and advocacy leads to the protégé's self-belief, self-confidence, empowerment, and achievement—the self-fulfilling prophecy. When this occurs, protégés develop their potential and gain strength and confidence to achieve at high levels. As we know, success is not a random act. "It arises out of a predictable and powerful set of circumstances and opportunities" (Gladwell, 2008). These circumstances and opportunities include having mentors who believe in us, expect us to succeed, champion our work, and inevitably have a profound effect on who we are and what we become and achieve. **The bottom line: Mentoring is truly a transformative act.**

Reciprocal sharing is an essential element of mentoring. If you have been mentored, you have an obligation to give back the gift of mentoring to others, be they students, peers, or even expert colleagues. If you have experienced the power of belief and expectation from Pygmalion–Mentors, you are in a strategic position to mentor others in that framework. If you have had the privilege of mentoring in your life, you know how it works. Then it becomes your privilege and obligation to be a good mentor–leader. Here is where your Mentor Intelligence enters the picture. Reflect on the three components of Mentor Intelligence, and review your intentions and behaviors to mentor your colleagues and students. Each component will contribute to your growing confidence. As you activate your Mentor Intelligence, you will energize others in a dynamic legacy of mentoring.

- Do you have a **mentoring mentality** about helping others grow and develop?
- Do you see students and your nursing colleagues through a **mentoring lens**—of wanting to help and support them through the mentoring process?
- Do you create a **mentoring momentum** of creating and sustaining mentor relationships?

FAST FACTS in a NUTSHELL

- One person's beliefs and expectations have a powerful effect on another person's beliefs and behaviors that acts as a "self-fulfilling prophecy."

Continued

Continued

- When nurses *believe* in each other, and *expect* and *support* each other's achievement and success, they are serving as transformational Pygmalion–Mentors.
- As a Pygmalion–Mentor–Leader, you will develop the three competencies of Mentor Intelligence: mentoring lens, mentoring mentality, and mentoring momentum.

10

Top Ten Tips to Raise Your Mentor Intelligence

In the final analysis, the true road to success lies not in a person's molecular structure, but in developing the most productive attitudes and identifying magnificent external resources.

—David Shenk (2010)

INTRODUCTION

Mentor Intelligence is a valuable source of excellence that will enhance your unique personal gifts. Mentors are a "magnificent external resource." They are the spark and fuel for your professional and life journey. Becoming a successful competent professional nurse is a lifelong process. Mentor Intelligence will help you attract essential support and you in turn will mentor others. This chapter provides 10 tips for raising your Mentor Intelligence.

In this chapter, you will learn:

1. About Mentor Intelligence as a source of excellence
2. Ten tips for raising your Mentor Intelligence

"STAR POWER" REQUIRES MENTOR INTELLIGENCE

You have learned that a combination of many factors, internal and external, influence life and work success—for better or worse. These multiple factors provide the raw materials that contribute to a person's potential for achievement and superior competence. Factors that propel people to rise to "star power" include parentage, protection, hard work, motivation, perseverance, and opportunities (Gladwell, 2008). In order to perform successfully in a complex profession like nursing, there are beginning threshold requirements such as intellectual intelligence (IQ) and specialized knowledge and skills. Further, it is thought that working at a high level of excellence in one's field requires emotional intelligence. In fact, it has been widely documented that the lack of emotional intelligence prevents the freeing of other "intelligences."

In this book I have suggested that another form of intelligence—Mentor Intelligence—is an invaluable contributor to excellence and leadership development. Possessing this form of intelligence places you in a position of strength to obtain the necessary support to reach "the stars." You can be a good nurse if you are "smart," motivated, and work hard to improve your skills. However, the lack of Mentor Intelligence presents major impediments in developing one's full potential to the highest level. The nurse who doesn't have mentoring is handicapped due to lack of support, access, and information.

This book has described the three competencies of Mentor Intelligence: (1) possessing a mentoring mentality, (2) seeing yourself and others through a mentoring lens, and (3) creating a mentoring momentum. Each of these will make a substantial contribution to giving and receiving the gift of mentoring with your expert and peer mentors. The good news is that you can raise your Mentor Intelligence through knowledge, intention, and strategic actions. **The bottom line: Reach for the stars— the highest level of achievement that you are capable of—and find fulfillment as an excellent professional nurse.**

TOP TEN TIPS FOR RAISING YOUR MENTOR INTELLIGENCE

1. **Cultivate the three ingredients of Mentor Intelligence.** Try regularly to enhance your *mentoring mentality* through knowledge and awareness; see yourself and others through a *mentoring lens*; and create a *mentoring momentum* in your relationships. Be an eager and "attractive" protégé—proactive in finding mentors for yourself—as many as possible. Be a mentor to as many students and colleagues as you can—sharing with those who show you by their attitudes and behaviors that they are desirous of being helped with your involvement.

2. **Practice your profession in a culture of mentorship and collegiality.** Seek employment in an organization that values learning and promotes the development of its members. Work in an organization that acknowledges and meets the special mentoring needs of students and nurses in the beginning and evolving stages of their careers. By your own example and attitude, help to create the value and expectation of mentoring. Do not accept intimidation, lateral violence, or any form of disrespectful collegial behaviors where you work and study. Reject "tormenting" behaviors and foster mentoring behaviors. Help to create healthy work environments and "places of realized potential." Offer everyday the gift of compassion and caring to your colleagues.

3. **Invest in yourself and others through mentor bonds.** Generously give and receive the gift of mentoring with your colleagues. Remember that every nurse and every student deserves to be mentored and that they have the privilege and obligation to mentor each other. Feel the pride and power in nursing's unique contributions to society. Advocate strongly for the excellence of your and your colleagues' work that showcases nursing's value to patients and families. Help to "grow" the talents of nurses who reflect your professional values and holistic "ways of knowing" nursing.

4. **Expect great things of yourself and your colleagues.** Believe in yourself and others—and expect success and achievement. Act as a Pygmalion–Mentor. Remember that your beliefs and expectations have a powerful influence on your colleagues' and students' behaviors, which creates a self-fulfilling prophecy. Have faith in

your nursing colleagues, and be their champion and advocate. Belief and advocacy promotes individual and collective confidence and motivation to be the "best and brightest."

5. **Network, network, network.** Remember that networking is both an attitude and a way of life. Networking and learning are synonymous. Network everyday— using both face-to-face and electronic avenues. If you associate with "connected" people, you will be connected. If you network, you are visible. Activate networking at every meeting, conference, class, social gathering—wherever you are and wherever you go. Share your contacts and information, and generously help others to build their networks. Be a mentoring presence with others. Join professional associations. Always carry business cards and have an up-to-date resume and print and electronic address books—your passport to many career milestones.

6. **Sharpen your communication skills and your message.** Practice and fine-tune your listening, speaking, and writing skills. Your message is composed of your body language, voice, words, and communication style. Make certain that your total "communication package" works for you. Get feedback from mentors about your effectiveness as a communicator. Be certain that your telephonic and electronic messages and addresses are "to the point" and "professional." Be careful about protecting your privacy and professionalism with online social networking.

7. **Become a mentor–leader.** Remember that a good leader, even a novice leader, can teach, mentor, and develop others. "Polishing gifts" of your colleagues and team

members through mentoring will give you the enormous satisfaction and joy of helping them reach their potential and achieve excellence. Remember that you will also be inspired and taught by the people you mentor. As your life has been changed by mentors, you in turn can influence other's lives through your mentoring connections. Remember that you will be inspired and taught by the people you mentor. Identify yourself as a mentor–leader through your attitudes and actions, and pass the torch of success to others as you grow in your professional career. Remember to honor and thank your mentors! They will appreciate your recognition and respect.

8. **Be a "forever" student of mentoring, and develop the art of mentoring others.** Learn how mentorship works, and practice refining your mentor skills in your daily interactions. Use the word "mentor" in your thinking and communication with others. Reflect on relationships with your mentors and protégés, and how you can improve these mentor bonds. To develop your professional power and become an expert nurse, obtain the highest academic credentials. Do excellent work for your patients and families, and inspire and motivate students and colleagues to do likewise.

9. **Be a "mentor groupie."** Your network is the people you know and "hang out" with. Your group networks are a major influence in your career. Become a member of professional associations and assume leadership roles. Professional group membership is a vehicle for mentors and protégés to find each other. Being a consummate group member will provide you with

multiple opportunities for learning, leadership development, and specialty skill enhancement. Organize a mentor program at your school or workplace. Start your own Peer Mentoring Group with several colleagues, and meet regularly to share information, problem-solve, and to coach each other. Create a board of mentors, consisting of a variety of mentors, who will support your diverse needs and interests.

10. **Discover your passion, your "fire"—set your goals—and find your motivation.** Examine your dreams and goals. Discover what "fires you up" and brings you joy—what motivates you to work long and hard—with pleasure. Both careful planning and serendipity can fuel your passions and advance your goals. Find heroes—people who inspire you to reach higher than you ever imagined. Aspire to work at the "top of your game." Find the pleasure of learning under the gaze of an interested mentor. Give yourself the joy of mentoring with someone who wants to grow with you.

FAST FACTS in a NUTSHELL

- Mentor Intelligence is a major source of excellence, along with intellectual intelligence, emotional intelligence, and educational preparation.
- Raise your Mentor Intelligence, and you will be the giver and recipient of the gift of mentoring in your life and career path.
- Reach for the stars and gain power to scale the mountains.

Mentor Lessons appear to us through legend, literature, life experiences, narratives, film, and research. *The Goose Story* has mentor lessons that tell us what we need to do as we "fly" through life. Geese fly thousands of miles every year. They can move hundreds of miles in a day. They are truly one of the wonders of our world. And they do it by honking encouragement and cheering each other on every step of the way (Blanchard & Bowles, 1998). Here is the Lesson of the Goose as an extra "tip" for success in your mentoring journey through life.

The Goose Story

Next fall, when you see Geese heading South for the winter—flying along in V formation—you might consider what science has discovered as to why they fly that way:

As each bird flaps its Wings, it creates an Uplift for the bird immediately Following.

By flying in V formation, the Whole Flock adds at least 71 percent greater Flying Range than if each bird Flew on its Own.

People who share a common direction and sense of community can get where they are going more quickly and easily because they are traveling on the thrust of one another.

When a goose Falls out of Formation, it suddenly feels the Drag and Resistance of trying to go it alone—and quickly gets back into formation to take Advantage of the Lifting Power of the bird in front.

If we have as much sense as a goose, we will stay in formation with those who are headed the same way we are.

When the Head Goose gets tired, it rotates back in the Wing and another goose flies Point.

It is sensible to take turns doing demanding jobs with people.

Geese honk from behind to Encourage those up Front to keep up their Speed.

What do we say when we honk from behind?

Finally—when a goose gets Sick, or it is wounded by Gunshot and falls out of Formation, two other Geese fall out with that goose and follow it down to lend Help and Protection. They stay with the Fallen Goose until it is able to Fly, or until it dies; and only then do they launch out on their own, or with another Formation to catch up with their Group.

If we have the sense of a goose we will stand by each other like that.

—Dr. Harry Clarke Hoyes (1992)

Postscript

During my career journey, special colleagues and I have shared the magic of mentoring. One of these nursing colleagues has been a continuing source of inspiration and influence. Dr. Ruth Watson Lubic is a renowned international nurse midwife and the first nursing recipient of the MacArthur Foundation "genius award" for her role in contributing to a better world. Ruth is a powerful role model, innovator, and advocate—a true hero and nursing leader extraordinaire. I deeply admire her passion for her patients (always first and foremost in her thoughts and actions), her colleagues, and her profession. She is a reminder of the power of one person to make a difference in a single life and thousands of lives. Ruth does "her magic" with unwavering determination. She once gave me her *Principles for a Successful Professional Life*, which I have given to numerous students and nurses. I share Dr. Lubic's "secrets of success" with you on the following page as a special gift on your journey to career success and happiness. Good Luck!

Principles for a Successful Professional Life

Ruth Watson Lubic, RN, CNM, EDD, FAAN, FACNM

Begin with the needs of the people you serve.

Take care of all the people of the nation.

Trust your caring instincts.

Learn to tolerate uncertainty and ambiguity.

Choose your colleagues for their caring philosophy, not just their preparation.

Be aware that the medical model has failed to serve all the people of the nation.

Avoid anger—it consumes energy and clouds your vision.

Avoid bitterness against opponents, a useless distraction.

Value the giving and receiving of truth.

Strengthen your sense of humor—it can neutralize opposition and brighten the darkest days.

Recognize the importance of persistence.

Base a design for change on the best science possible and then test your performance.

Overcome the fears associated with leadership.

Remember: The people you serve are your strength. Listen to them. You will be rewarded.

Source: Adapted from Ruth W. Lubic, 2010, with permission.

Appendices

Appendix A: Personal Mentor Action Plan

Vision and Goals	Mentoring Strategies	Implementation Activities	Mentoring Outcomes

Appendix B: Resources for Collective Mentoring and Networking

Collective mentoring is "on the move" with many exciting initiatives. "Collective mentoring is about the process of working together to extend nursing's solidarity of activists. It also is about recognizing that new, even inexperienced, voices can contribute to the development of the most seasoned mentors" (Leavitt, Chaffee, & Vance, 2007). Getting connected through collective and group mentoring avenues is a must for nurses' career development, lifelong learning, and leadership opportunities. The special benefits of various types of collective mentoring simply cannot be overemphasized.

Professional associations are a major resource for collective mentoring and networking. They provide special membership services to students, generalist and specialty nurses, nursing leaders, nursing alumni, and nurses in special interest groups, such as international, multicultural, and racial-ethnic. Empowered nurses have joined together to build these associations, and there are literally hundreds of them. Every professional nurse should join at least two or three associations for mentorship, networking, and collegial activities that support professional practice and leadership development. Membership and activism in professional associations offers these collective benefits:

- Priceless mentoring with peer and expert colleagues
- Networking: in person and online
- Educational opportunities: meetings, conferences, conventions, scholarships, and research support
- Information: journals, newsletters, booklets, audio-visuals, Web sites, Webinars, Facebook, Twitter, Flickr, blogs, discussion boards
- Leadership training and development: fellowships, programs, committee service, office holding, volunteer activities
- Having a voice in professional, political, and health policy issues
- Participation in decision making about nursing and health-care matters

A Sample of Mentor Resources in Nursing Associations:

- Academy of Medical-Surgical Nurses. Nurses Nurturing Nurses (N3) Mentoring Program, consisting of two formats: online and hospital-based. www.amsn.org
- American Academy of Nurse Practitioners. FAANP Mentoring Program. www.aanp.org
- American Association of Critical Care Nurses. www.aacn.org
- Minnesota Nurses Association. Commission on Education. *Mentoring Relationships* (2002). St. Paul, MN. www.mnnurses.org

- International Council of Nurses (ICN). www.icn.org
- National Association of Hispanic Nurses. www.nahn.org
- National Black Nurses Association. www.nbna.org
- National Student Nurses' Association. *Mentoring. The experience of a lifetime* (2005). Video and DVD. Brooklyn, NY. www.nsna.org
- Oncology Nursing Society. *Mentorship: Our commitment to our future* (2001). Video. www.oncology nursingsociety.org
- Sigma Theta Tau International. Honor Society in Nursing. Chiron Mentored Leadership Development Program. www.nursingsociety.org/mentoring
- Transcultural Nursing Society and Regional Chapters. www.tcns.org

Other Mentoring Associations:

- International Mentoring Association. www.mentoring-association.org
- Triple Creek Associates, Inc. Web-based and e-mentoring—Webinars, Podcasts, newsletter, *Masterful Mentoring.* www.3creek.com

For other mentoring programs, search online for "mentoring programs."

Web Resources:

- American Nurses Association: http://nursingworld.org

- GEM-Nursing: An online mentoring resource program. www.gem-nursing.org
- Mentoring in Nursing search engines: www.info.com/mentoring
- Mentor Match: www.mentormatch.com
- Nurse LinkUp: www.nurselinkup.com/
- *Nursing Spectrum and Nurse Week*: www.nurse.com

References & Bibliography

Albom, M. (1997). *Tuesdays with Morrie: An old man, a young man, and life's greatest lesson.* New York: Doubleday.

Allen, D. W. (1998). How nurses become leaders: Perceptions and beliefs about leadership development. *Journal of Nursing Administration, 28*(9), 15–20.

American Nurses Association. (2001). *Code of ethics for nurses with interpretive statements.* Silver Spring, MD: Nursesbooks.org.

American Nurses Association. (2010). *Nursing's social policy statement: The essence of the profession.* Silver Spring, MD: Nursesbooks.org.

American Nurses Association. (2004). *Nursing: Scope and standards of practice* (1st ed.). Silver Spring, MD: Nursesbooks.org.

American Nurses Association. (2010). *Nursing: Scope and standards of practice* (2nd ed.). Silver Spring, MD: Nursesbooks.org.

Arnoldussen, B. (2007). *First year nurse* (2nd ed.). New York: Kaplan Publishing.

Benner, P. (1984). *From novice to expert: Excellence and power in clinical nursing practice.* Menlo Park, CA: Addison-Wesley.

Billings, D., & Kowalski, K. (2006). Journaling: A strategy for developing reflective practitioners. *The Journal of Continuing Education in Nursing, 37*(3), 104–105.

Blanchard, K., & Bowles, S. (1998). *Gung ho!* New York: William Morrow & Company.

Blanchard, K., Carlos, J., & Randolph, A. (1996). *Empowerment takes more than a minute.* San Francisco: Berrett-Koehler.

Brucker, J., & Charlie, M. (1998). Interview of a teacher–mentor and student protégé. In C. Vance, & R. Olson (Eds.), *The mentor connection in nursing* (pp. 60–66). New York: Springer.

Campbell, L., Gilbert, M., & Lausten, G. (2010). *Clinical coach for nursing excellence.* Philadelphia: FA Davis.

Casey, K., Fink, R., Krugman, M., & Propst, J. (2004). The graduate nurse experience. *Journal of Nursing Administration, 34*(6), 303–311.

Chitty, K. K., & Black, B. B. (2007). *Professional nursing: Concepts & challenges* (5th ed.). St. Louis: Saunders Elsevier.

Christakis, N. A., & Fowler, J. H. (2009). *Connected: The surprising power of our social networks and how they shape our lives.* New York: Little, Brown.

Collins, E., & Scott, P. (1978). Everyone who makes it has a mentor. *Harvard Business Review, 56*(4), 89–101.

Collins, N. W. (1983). *Professional women and their mentors.* Englewood Cliffs, NJ: Prentice-Hall.

Coyle, D. (2009). *The talent code.* New York: Bantam Dell.

Daloz, L. A. (1986). *Effective teaching and mentoring: Realizing the transformational power of adult learning experiences.* San Francisco: Jossey-Bass.

Daloz, L. A. (1999). *Mentor: Guiding the journey of adult learners.* San Francisco: Jossey-Bass.

Dalton, G., Thompson, P., & Price, R. (1977, Summer). The four stages of professional careers. *Organizational Dynamics, 6,* 19–42.

Dalton, M. (2010). *The Hollywood curriculum: Teachers in the movies.* New York: Peter Lang.

Darling, D. (2003). *The networking survival guide: Get the success you want by tapping into the people you know.* New York: McGraw-Hill.

DeLong, T., Gabarro, J., & Lees, R. (2008). Why mentoring matters in a hyper-competitive world. *Howard Business Review, 8*(1), 115–121.

De Pree, M. (1989). *Leadership is an art* (2nd ed.). New York: Doubleday.

De Pree, M. (1992). *Leadership jazz.* New York: Dell.

De Pree, M. (1997). *Leading without power: Finding hope in serving community.* San Francisco: Jossey-Bass.

Dyess, S., & Sherman, R. (2009). The first year of practice: New graduate nurses' transition and learning needs. *The Journal of Continuing Education in Nursing, 40*(9), 403–410.

Eden, D. (1990). *Pygmalion in management: Productivity as a self-fulfilling prophecy.* Lexington, MA: Lexington Books.

Ensher, E., & Murphy, S. (2005). *Power mentoring: How successful mentors and protégés get the most out of their relationships.* San Francisco: Jossey-Bass.

Fawcett, D. (2002). Mentoring—What it is and how to make it work. *AORN Journal, 75*(5), 950–954.

Felton, G. (1978). On women, networks, patronage and sponsorship. *Image: Journal of Nursing Scholarship, 10*(3), 58–59.

Finkelman, A., & Kenner, C. (2010). *Professional nursing concepts: Competencies for quality leadership.* Sudbury, MA: Jones & Bartlett.

Gladwell, M. (2000). *The tipping point: How little things can make a big difference.* New York: Little, Brown.

Gladwell, M. (2008). *Outliers: The story of success.* New York: Little, Brown.

Goleman, D. (1995). *Emotional intelligence.* New York: Bantam.

Goleman, D. (1998). *Working with emotional intelligence.* New York: Bantam Dell.

Goleman, D., Boyatzis, R., & McKee, A. (2002). *Primal leadership: Learning to lead with emotional intelligence.* Boston: Harvard Business School Press.

Greenleaf, R. K. (1977). *Servant leadership: A journey into the nature of legitimate power and greatness.* New York: Paulist Press.

Griffin, M. (2004). Teaching cognitive rehearsal as a shield for lateral violence: An intervention for newly licensed nurses. *The Journal of Continuing Education in Nursing, 35*(6), 257–263.

Grossman, S. C. (2007). *Mentoring in nursing: A dynamic and collaborative process.* New York: Springer.

Grossman, S. C., & Valiga, T. M. (2009). *The new leadership challenge: Creating the future of nursing* (3rd ed.). Philadelphia: FA Davis.

Hall, D., & Rosenberg, C. (2009). *Get connected*. Madison, WI: Entrepreneurial Press.

Homer (1967). *The odyssey* (A. Cook, Trans.). New York: Norton.

Hoyes, H. C. (1992). The goose story. *ARCS News, 7*(1), 6.

Huang, C. A., & Lynch, J. (1995). *Mentoring: The Tao of giving and receiving wisdom*. New York: HarperSanFrancisco.

Johnson, W. B., & Ridley, C. R. (2004). *The elements of mentoring*. New York: Palgrave Macmillan.

Joint Commission (2008). *Behaviors that undermine a culture of safety*. Sentinel Event Alert #40. Retrieved July 9, 2008, from http://www.jointcommission.org/SentinelEvents/SentinelEventAlert/sea_40.htm

Kegan, R. (1982). *The evolving self: Problem and process in human development*. Cambridge, MA: Harvard University Press.

Laschinger, H. K., Finegan, J., & Wilk, P. (2009). New graduate burnout: The impact of professional practice environment, workplace civility, and empowerment. *Nursing Economics, 27*(6), 377–383.

Leavitt, J. K., Chaffee, M., & Vance, C. (2007). Learning the ropes of policy, politics, and advocacy. In D. Mason, J. K. Leavitt, & M. Chaffee (Eds.), *Policy and politics in nursing and health care* (5th ed.). St. Louis, MO: Saunders Elsevier.

Leavitt, J. K., & Mason, D. (1998). The good ol' girls and collective mentoring. In C. Vance, & R. Olson (Eds.), *The mentor connection in nursing* (pp. 160–162). New York: Springer.

Levitin, D. J. (2006). *This is your brain on music: The science of a human obsession*. New York: Dutton.

Livingston, J. S. (1988). Pygmalion in management. *Harvard Business Review Classic, September–October*, 121–130.

Lorentzon, M., & Brown, K. (2003). Florence Nightingale as "mentor of matrons": Correspondence with Rachel Williams at St. Mary's Hospital. *Journal of Nursing Management, 11*, 266–274.

Malone, B. (1998). Mentoring: A song of power. In C. Vance, & R. Olson (Eds.), *The mentor connection in nursing* (pp. 56–60). New York: Springer.

Mason, D. J. (2001). Of mentorship and scotch on the rocks. *American Journal of Nursing, 101*(7), 7.

Misner, I. R. (2008). *The 29% solution: 52 weekly networking success strategies.* Austin, TX: Greenleaf Book Group Press.

National Student Nurses' Association. (1996). *Resolution: In support of the promotion, awareness, and development of mentorship programs.* Retrieved from www.nsna.org/Publications/Resolutions. aspx

National Student Nurses' Association. (2001). *Resolution: In support of the prevention of workplace violence in health care settings through increased education and awareness.* Retrieved from www. nsna.org/Publications/Resolutions.aspx

National Student Nurses' Association. (2002). *Resolution: In support of encouraging peer mentorship programs to be incorporated into nursing curricula and/or student nurses associations.* Retrieved from www.nsna.org/Publications/Resolutions. aspx

National Student Nurses' Association. (2006). *Resolution: In support of increased advocacy for improved preceptor programs to create a robust workforce environment for the nursing profession.* Retrieved from www.nsna.org/Publications/Resolutions. aspx

National Student Nurses' Association. (2006). *Resolution: In support of professional workplace cultures and decreasing horizontal violence.* Retrieved from www.nsna.org/Publications/Resolutions. aspx

National Student Nurses' Association. (2010). *Resolution: In support of policy development and increased funding for research on lateral violence in nursing.* Retrieved from www.nsna.org/Publications/ Resolutions.aspx

New York State Education Department. (1972). *Education law, article 139: Nursing.* www.op.nyset.gov/nurse

Nightingale, F. (1881). Address. In M. Vicinus, & B. Nergaard (1990). *Ever yours, Florence Nightingale: Selected letters.* Cambridge, MA: Harvard University Press.

Olson, M. E. (2009). The "millennials": First year in practice. *Nursing Outlook, 57,* 10–17.

Olson, R., & Vance, C. (1993). *Mentorship in nursing: A collection of research abstracts with selected bibliographies—1977–1992.* Houston, TX: University of Texas Printing.

Olson, R., & Vance, C. (1998). Mentorship in nursing education. In K. A. Stevens (Ed.), *Review of research in nursing education* (Vol. 8). New York: National League for Nursing.

Pellico, L., Brewer, C., & Kovner, C. (2009). What newly licensed registered nurses have to say about their first experiences. *Nursing Outlook, 57,* 194–203.

Porter-O-Grady, P., & Malloch, K. (2007). *Quantum leadership: A resource for health care innovation* (2nd ed.). Sudbury, MA: Jones & Bartlett.

Reynolds, J. (2007). Negativity in the workplace. *American Journal of Nursing, 107,* 72D–72G.

Roche, J., Morsi, D., & Chandler, G. (2009). Testing a work empowerment–work relationship model to explain expertise in experienced acute care nurses. *The Journal of Nursing Administration, 39*(3), 115–122.

Salmon, M. E. (1998). Mentorship: A personal perspective. In C. Vance, & R. Olson (Eds.), *The mentor connection in nursing* (pp. 66–70). New York: Springer.

Schorr, T. (1979). Mentor remembered. *American Journal of Nursing, 79,* 65.

Shenk, D. (2010). *The genius in all of us: Why everything you've been told about genetics, talents, and IQ is wrong.* New York: Doubleday.

Simonton, D. K. (2009). *Genius 101.* New York: Springer.

Sinetar, M. (1998). *The mentor's spirit: Life lessons on leadership and the art of encouragement.* New York: St. Martin's Press.

Stanley, K., Martin, M., Michel, Y., Welton, J., & Nemeth, L. (2007). Examining lateral violence in the nursing workforce. *Issues in Mental Health Nursing, 28,* 1247–1265.

Thomas, S. P., & Burk, R. (2009). Junior nursing students' experiences of vertical violence during clinical rotations. *Nursing Outlook, 57,* 226–231.

Thomka, L. A. (2007). Mentoring and its impact on intellectual capital: Through the eyes of the mentee. *Nurse Administrative Quarterly, 31*(1), 22–26.

Vance, C. (1977). A group profile of contemporary influentials in American nursing (Doctoral dissertation, Teachers College, Columbia University, 1977). *Dissertation Abstracts International, 38,* 4734B.

Vance, C. (1982). The mentor connection. *Journal of Nursing Administration, 12*(4), 7–13.

Vance, C. (1999). Mentoring and networking—The student's perspective. In C. A. Andersen (Ed.), *Nursing student to nursing leader: The critical path to leadership development.* Albany, New York: Delmar.

Vance, C. (2001). The ABCs of mentoring. *Nursing Spectrum, 13*(4), 6.

Vance, C. (2001). The value of mentoring. *Imprint, 48*(2), 38–40.

Vance, C. (2002). Leader as mentor. *Nursing Leadership Forum, 7*(2), 83–90.

Vance, C. (2005). Leader as mentor. In H. Feldman, & M. Greenberg (Eds.), *Educating nurses for leadership.* New York: Springer.

Vance, C. (2007). Nurse mentoring: A key to retaining talent in the hospital. *Nursing Spectrum, March 16,* 12–13.

Vance, C. (2009). *The mentor as Pygmalion: Realizing potential through empowerment.* International Association of Mentoring. Annual convention.

Vance, C., & Olson, R. (1991). Mentorship. In J. Fitzpatrick, R. Taunton, & A. Jacox (Eds.), *Annual Review of Nursing Research* (Vol. 9, pp. 175–200). New York: Springer.

Vance, C., & Olson, R. (1998). *The mentor connection in nursing.* New York: Springer.

Wheatley, M. J. (1999). *Leadership and the new science: Discovering order in a chaotic world* (2nd ed.). San Francisco: Berrett-Koehler Publishers.

Wickman, F., & Sjodin, T. (1997). *Mentoring: The most obvious yet overlooked key to achieving more in life than you dreamed possible: A success guide for mentors and protégés.* New York: McGraw-Hill.

Zachary, L. J. (2005). *Creating a mentoring culture.* San Francisco: Jossey-Bass.

Zachary, L. J. (2009). *The mentee's guide: Making mentoring work for you.* San Francisco: Jossey-Bass.

Zey, M. G. (1984). *The mentor connection.* Homewood, IL: Dow Jones-Irwin.

Index

Printed in the United States
By Bookmasters